Haldimand County Public Library
CALEDONIA BRANCH
100 Haddington St. Unit 2
Caledonia ON N3W 2N4

JAN 0 3 2006

FEB 2 7 2006

MAY 0 4 2007

MAY 1 1 2007

OCT 1 8 2011

MAR 2 7 2013

APR 1 6 2014

Drug Therapy and Cognitive Disorders

Psychiatric Disorders
Drugs and Psychology for the Mind and Body

Drug Therapy and Adjustment Disorders

Drug Therapy and Anxiety Disorders

Drug Therapy and Cognitive Disorders

Drug Therapy and Childhood and Adolescent Disorders

Drug Therapy and Dissociative Disorders

Drug Therapy and Eating Disorders

Drug Therapy and Impulse Control Disorders

Drug Therapy for Mental Disorders Caused by a Medical Condition

Drug Therapy and Mood Disorders

Drug Therapy and Obsessive-Compulsive Disorder

Drug Therapy and Personality Disorders

Drug Therapy and Postpartum Disorders

Drug Therapy and Premenstrual Disorders

Drug Therapy and Psychosomatic Disorders

Drug Therapy and Schizophrenia

Drug Therapy and Sexual Disorders

Drug Therapy and Sleep Disorders

Drug Therapy and Substance-Related Disorders

The FDA and Psychiatric Drugs: How a Drug Is Approved

Psychiatric Disorders: Drugs and Psychology for the Mind and Body

Drug Therapy and Cognitive Disorders

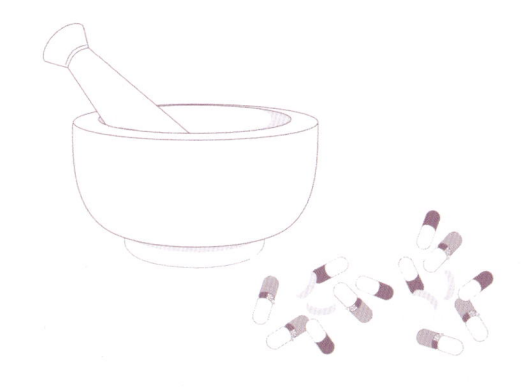

BY SHERRY BONNICE AND CAROLYN HOARD

MASON CREST PUBLISHERS
PHILADELPHIA

Mason Crest Publishers Inc.
370 Reed Road
Broomall, Pennsylvania 19008
(866) MCP-BOOK (toll free)

Copyright © 2004 by Mason Crest Publishers. All rights reserved. No part of this publication may be reproduced or transmitted in any form or by any means, electronic or mechanical, including photocopying, recording, taping, or any information storage and retrieval system, without permission from the publisher.

First printing
1 2 3 4 5 6 7 8 9 10

Bonnice, Sherry, 1956-
Drug therapy and cognitive disorders / by Sherry Bonnice and Carolyn Hoard.
v. cm.—(Psychiatric disorders: drugs and psychology for the mind and body)
Includes bibliographical references and index.
Contents: Defining cognitive disorders, including Alzheimer's—The history of drugs' role in cognitive disorders—How do the drugs work?—Treatment description—Case histories—Risks and side effects—Alternative and supplementary treatments.
1. Cognition disorders—Chemotherapy—Juvenile literature. [1. Cognition disorders. 2. Mental illness.] I. Hoard, Carolyn. II. Title. III. Series.
RC553.C64B66 2004
616.89'18—dc21
2003005721

ISBN 1-59084-562-5
ISBN 1-59084-559-5 (series)

Design by Lori Holland.
Composition by Bytheway Publishing Services, Binghamton, New York.
Cover design by Benjamin Stewart.
Printed and bound in the Hashemite Kingdom of Jordan.

This book is meant to educate and should not be used as an alternative to appropriate medical care. Its creators have made every effort to ensure that the information presented is accurate—but it is not intended to substitute for the help and services of trained professionals.

Picture Credits:
Artville: pp. 105, 121. Autumn Libal: p. 50. Benjamin Stewart: pp. 49, 53, 62. Comstock: pp. 61, 70, 72, 74, 76, 119. Corbis: pp. 26, 29, 33, 54, 66, 78, 82, 92, 115, 116. Edward VanDeMark: p. 110. National Library of Medicine: p 76. PhotoDisc: pp. 10, 14, 44, 46, 57, 64, 80, 86, 89, 94, 97, 98, 102, 106, 112, 118, 122. Rubberball: pp. 17, 75, 90, 91, 108. Stockbyte: pp.12, 24, 58, 84, 101. The individuals in these images are models, and the images are for illustrative purposes only.

CONTENTS

Introduction	7
Foreword	9
1. Defining Cognitive Disorders, Including Alzheimer's	11
2. The History of Drugs' Role in Cognitive Disorders	27
3. How Do the Drugs Work?	47
4. Treatment Description	65
5. Case Histories	81
6. Risks and Side Effects	95
7. Alternative and Supplementary Treatments	109
Further Reading	124
For More Information	125
Index	127

INTRODUCTION

by Mary Ann Johnson

Teenagers have reason to be interested in psychiatric disorders and their treatment. Friends, family members, and even teens themselves may experience one of these disorders. Using scenarios adolescents will understand, this series explains various psychiatric disorders and the drugs that treat them.

Diagnosis and treatment of psychiatric disorders in children between six and eighteen years old are well studied and documented in the scientific journals. In 1998, Roberts and colleagues identified and reviewed fifty-two research studies that attempted to identify the overall prevalence of child and adolescent psychiatric disorders. Estimates of prevalence in this review ranged from one percent to nearly 51 percent. Various other studies have reported similar findings. Needless to say, many children and adolescents are suffering from psychiatric disorders and are in need of treatment.

Many children have more than one psychiatric disorder, which complicates their diagnoses and treatment plans. Psychiatric disorders often occur together. For instance, a person with a sleep disorder may also be depressed; a teenager with attention-deficit/hyperactivity disorder (ADHD) may also have a substance-use disorder. In psychiatry, we call this comorbidity. Much research addressing this issue has led to improved diagnosis and treatment.

The most common child and adolescent psychiatric disorders are anxiety disorders, depressive disorders, and ADHD. Sleep disorders, sexual disorders, eating disorders, substance-abuse disorders, and psychotic disorders are also quite common. This series has volumes that address each of these disorders.

Major depressive disorders have been the most commonly diagnosed mood disorders for children and adolescents. Researchers don't agree as to how common mania and bipolar disorder are in children. Some experts believe that manic episodes in children and adolescents are under diagnosed. Many times, a mood disturbance may occur with another psychiatric disorder. For instance, children with ADHD may also be depressed. ADHD is just one psychiatric disorder that is a major health concern for children, adolescents, and adults. Studies of ADHD have reported prevalence rates among children that range from two to 12 percent.

Failure to understand or seek treatment for psychiatric disorders puts children and young adults at risk of developing substance-use disorders. For example, recent research indicates that those with ADHD who were treated with medication were 85 percent less likely to develop a substance-use disorder. Results like these emphasize the importance of timely diagnosis and treatment.

Early diagnosis and treatment may prevent these children from developing further psychological problems. Books like those in this series provide important information, an important first step toward increased awareness of psychological disorders; knowledge and understanding can shed light on even the most difficult subject. These books should never, however, be viewed as a substitute for professional consultation. Psychiatric testing and an evaluation by a licensed professional is recommended to determine the needs of the child or adolescent and to establish an appropriate treatment plan.

FOREWORD

by Donald Esherick

We live in a society filled with technology—from computers surfing the Internet to automobiles operating on gas and batteries. In the midst of this advanced society, diseases, illnesses, and medical conditions are treated and often cured with the administration of drugs, many of which were unknown thirty years ago. In the United States, we are fortunate to have an agency, the Food and Drug Administration (FDA), which monitors the development of new drugs and then determines whether the new drugs are safe and effective for use in human beings.

When a new drug is developed, a pharmaceutical company usually intends that drug to treat a single disease or family of diseases. The FDA reviews the company's research to determine if the drug is safe for use in the population at large and if it effectively treats the targeted illnesses. When the FDA finds that the drug is safe and effective, it approves the drug for treating that specific disease or condition. This is called the labeled indication.

During the routine use of the drug, the pharmaceutical company and physicians often observe that a drug treats other medical conditions besides what is indicated in the labeling. While the labeling will not include the treatment of the particular condition, a physician can still prescribe the drug to a patient with this disease. This is known as an unlabeled or off-label indication. This series contains information about both the labeled and off-label indication of psychiatric drugs.

I have reviewed the books in this series from the perspective of the pharmaceutical industry and the FDA, specifically focusing on the labeled indications, uses, and known side effects of these drugs. Further information can be found on the FDA's Web page (www.FDA.gov).

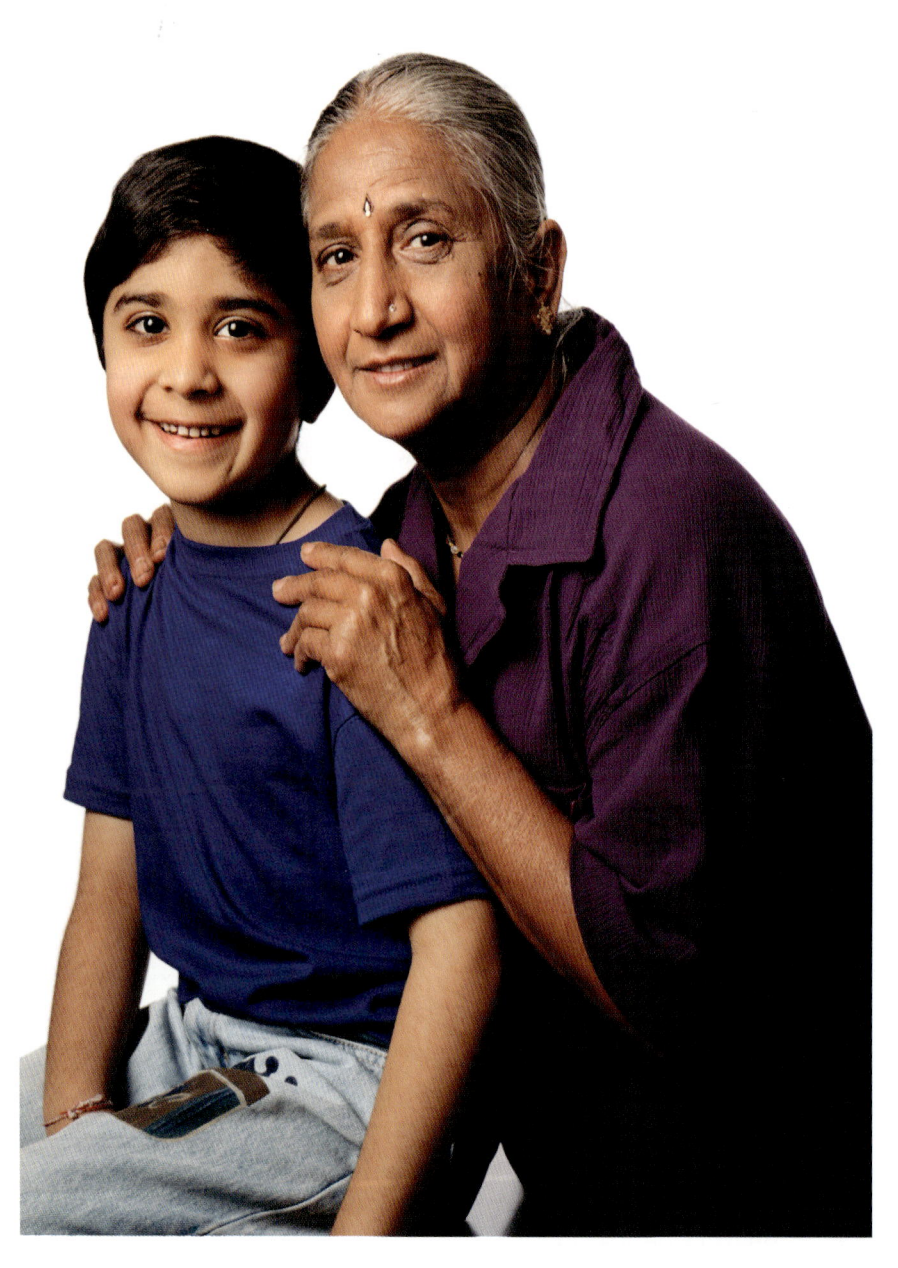

Grandparents can be a source of comfort and joy in a young person's life. When an older generation suffers memory loss, however, it can cause the entire family pain and confusion.

1 | Defining Cognitive Disorders, Including Alzheimer's

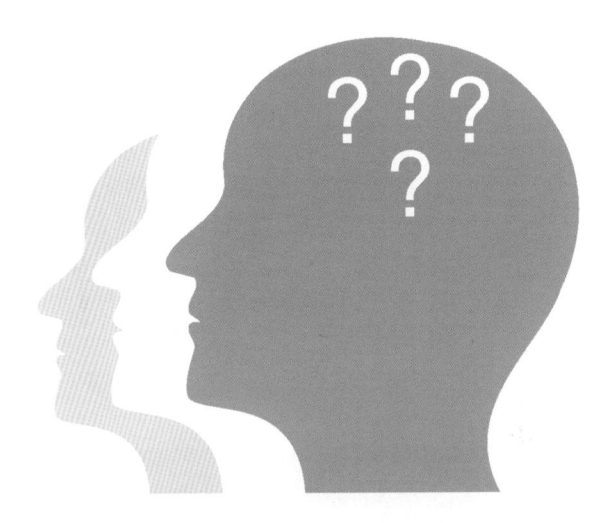

My dear grandchildren,

As I write to you today, some of you are young adults, while others of you are still babies. All of you have brought such joy into my life—you've changed me forever! I'm so glad you've been a part of my life—and that I've had the chance to be a part of yours.

As you continue to grow, I look forward to more times together—but I also know that the years will bring changes, as life brings you new opportunities. I've always looked forward to watching you at all the special events that mark your growth—concerts, sporting events, graduations, and yes, even weddings. I wanted to be a part of all your special times—but sometimes life brings other changes that aren't as easy. That's why I want to write to you now and tell you some things that will probably change for our family.

12 | CHAPTER 1

> **GLOSSARY**
>
> **cognitive:** Involving perception and thought processes.

You older children are aware I have a health problem that will probably affect the way I act toward you in the future. It will not change my heart or my feelings of love for each of you, but my behavior may seem a little "weird" at times. While you older ones can understand more of what may be happening to me, the younger ones will wonder why I act differently sometimes. I want to explain now, while I still can, so that when you're older you can read this and understand.

I have been diagnosed with a disease called mild cognitive impairment (MCI). Researchers believe that this is the beginning phase of a disease called Alzheimer's disease, which affects memory and other **cognitive** *functions. Although every patient who experiences a cognitive disorder is different, many patients have something in common.*

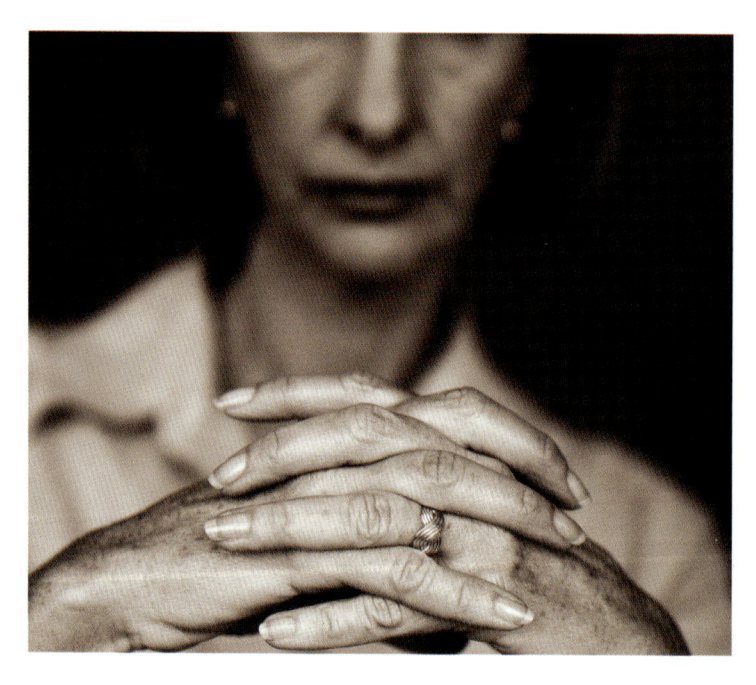

When a person's cognitive functions are impaired, she may feel as though she is forced to sit on the sidelines of life.

You're always saying to me, "Nana, I already told you that!" I know I ask you the same question over and over again—but I really can't remember. One of the crazy things about this disease is the strange way it affects my memory: I can still remember facts or conversations from a long time ago, but I can't remember what you said to me a few minutes ago. Sometimes people get angry because they think I'm not listening or paying attention when they talk to me. Please understand that I'm trying desperately to listen and remember—but my brain just won't cooperate. You've probably noticed I take a lot of notes; I write things down so I can help my memory a bit. I do this because I have learned that with the help of the notes I take I can piece together some conversations or facts. Just talking with the people I love the most has turned into such hard work!

You may also notice that sometimes I seem very tired and not much fun. That happens because struggling to remember the ordinary details of life takes such energy, that I get physically and mentally drained trying to keep up with everything going on around me. Sometimes I also get depressed and I just want to give up. But I have decided I don't want to lose touch with you, my precious ones, so I plan to keep writing you these "Notes from Nana" while I still can, so you will better understand what is happening to me as an individual and to other people who have this disease.

Love,
Nana Carolyn

Carolyn is in the early stages of Alzheimer's disease, a type of cognitive disorder classified as dementia that is characterized by a general loss of intellectual function. Dementia impairs the memory, judgment, and abstract thinking. The result of these changes may include altered personality, a gradual loss of memory, a lessoning in the ability to reason,

14 | CHAPTER 1

GLOSSARY

central nervous system: *The part of the nervous system that consists of the brain and spinal cord.*

difficulty in learning new things, and a decline in normal, everyday functioning. Although dementia may be caused by a variety of conditions, Alzheimer's disease is one of the most common. Some others include ***central nervous system*** (CNS) infection; vascular dementia, which is a disorder caused by a decrease in the blood flow to the brain; brain trauma or tumors; Pick's disease; Creutzfeldt-Jakob disease; pernicious anemia; folic acid deficiency; Wernicke Korsakoff syndrome; normal pressure hydrocephalus; and neurological diseases such as Huntington's disease, multiple sclerosis, and Parkinson's disease.

Carolyn is not yet experiencing dementia itself; instead, she has been diagnosed with a milder version, MCI, which manifests itself with signs of memory loss abnormal for her age. People like Carolyn may also have some problems with the chores and tasks involved with normal daily life. Although researchers have no absolute proof that MCI leads

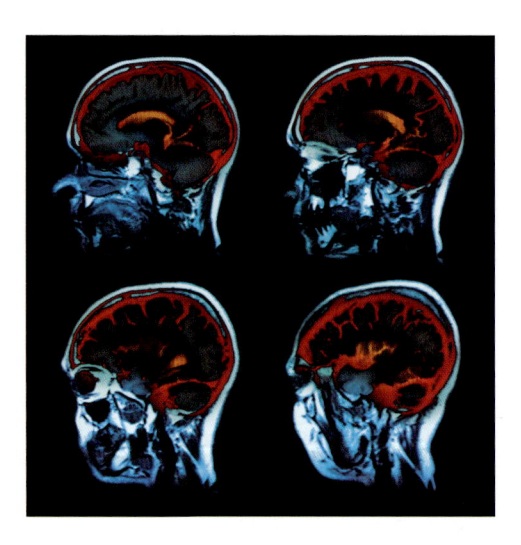

When a person has Alzheimer's disease, brain cells may be destroyed.

Defining Cognitive Disorders, Including Alzheimer's

> ### Kinds of Cognitive Disorders
> - delirium: a change in consciousness and thinking that develops over a short period of time.
> - dementia: includes multiple cognitive defects, including memory impairment.
> - amnestic disorder: memory loss without any other cognitive impairment.

to Alzheimer's, studies show that more than 80 percent of the patients who have MCI develop Alzheimer's disease within ten years. The evidence is fairly clear that many of those diagnosed with MCI are really in the early stages of this devastating disease.

In Alzheimer's disease, brain cells are destroyed, first in the area of the brain that controls memory and thinking and eventually in other brain areas that control other functions. The disease is progressive, which means that the patient will gradually get worse.

One of the most common early symptoms of Alzheimer's is a growing loss of memory; usually this involves short-term memory, the recollection of those things that happened within the last few minutes or the last few hours. This means the patient may forget what day or month it is. Even if someone tells her the date, within a few minutes, she will already have forgotten. The same person, however, may remember in detail things that happened forty-five years ago at her senior prom.

As with other dementias, symptoms include problems with reasoning or judgment, disorientation, difficulty in learning anything new, loss of language skills or the ability to communicate in any way, and the inability to do the everyday things that have been done for years. (For exam-

16 | CHAPTER 1

> According to the American Psychiatric Association's *Diagnostic and Statistical Manual, fourth edition* (the DSM-IV), a dementia involves:
>
> 1. memory impairment (impaired ability to learn new information or recall previously learned information)
> 2. one (or more) of the following cognitive disturbances:
>   a. aphasia (language disturbance)
>   b. apraxia (impaired ability to carry out motor activities despite intact motor function)
>   c. agnosia (failure to recognize or identify objects despite intact sensory functions)
>   d. disturbance in executive functioning (planning, organizing, sequencing, abstracting)

ple, some people with this disease may put their watch in the refrigerator and the lettuce in the bathroom.)

The disease can also cause personality changes. One woman whose mother suffered from Alzheimer's said, "I miss my mother. This is not the mother I grew up with. My mother's body is still alive, but my real mother is gone." Sometimes the changes produce anxiety; the individual may have a constant longing for home (even if she already is in her home), or she may long to be near one particular person. One woman, for instance, would sit sobbing, calling over and over for her husband—even though her husband was in a chair beside her bed. Sometimes a person with Alzheimer's becomes belligerent and angry. In other cases, the sufferer sees things that are not there or believes in a reality that does not exist.

One man remembers when he lived in an apartment next to his aging grandfather. His mother went every day to make sure her father had cooked meals and anything else he

Defining Cognitive Disorders, Including Alzheimer's | 17

needed. One day the grandson overheard his grandfather screaming at his mother. When the boy questioned his mother about it later, she merely shrugged. "Grandpa is old. Sometimes old people get like that." The young man was haunted by the sound of his grandfather's enraged bellows; he had always been such a quiet, gentle, and even-tempered man. As an adult today, the man wonders if his grandfather suffered from Alzheimer's; odds are good that he did.

Scientists do not completely understand what happens inside the brain when someone has Alzheimer's—but researchers are looking for the answers. In 1906, the German physician Dr. Alois Alzheimer was the first to study this tragic disease. During an *autopsy* of a woman who had suffered from dementia, Dr. Alzheimer noticed two abnormal structures: amyloid plaques, which are clumps of protein fragments that accumulate outside brain cells, and neu-

> **GLOSSARY**
>
> ***autopsy:*** *An examination of a body after death to determine the cause of death or the characteristics produced by disease.*

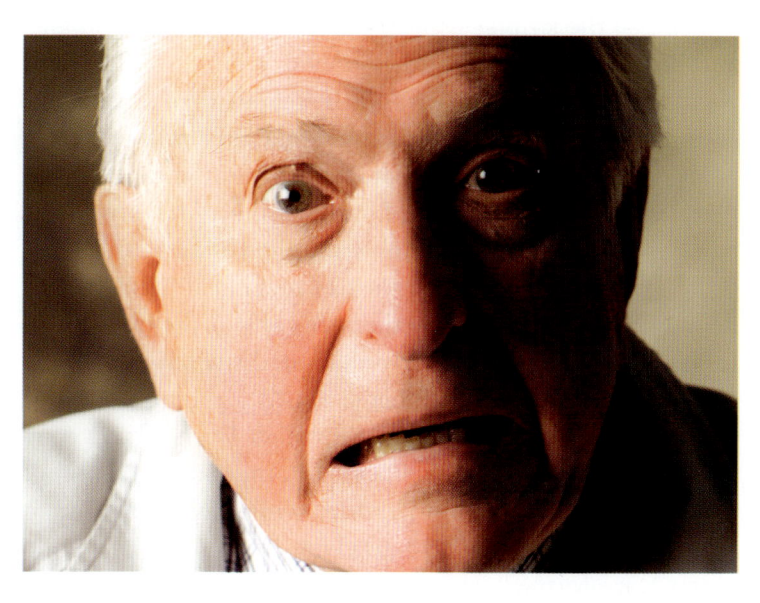

A person with a cognitive disorder may experience personality changes. This can be painful for family members.

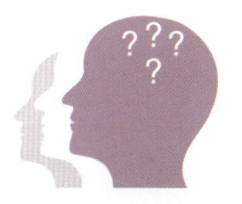

rofibrillary tangles, which are clumps of altered proteins inside the cells. Exactly what effect these clumps have on the brain is still unknown, but their presence is evidence of Alzheimer's disease.

The cerebral cortex, which is the outer portion of the brain, consisting of layers of nerve cells, is where thought processes take place, including conscious thoughts and language. In a normal brain, the nerve cells are arranged in an orderly way, but in an Alzheimer's patient's diseased brain, the cells become disorganized. It's as if nerve cells in the cerebral cortex and other regions of the brain were attacked by a deadly enemy. The formation of the neurofibrillary tangles and senile plaques begins to take over more and more of the brain, and as Alois Alzheimer first noticed, the cells are bunched up like a rope tied in knots. As the cells are attacked and killed, more and more of the symptoms become evident in the sufferer.

One of the strange aspects of the neurofibrillary tangles and senile plaques is that they only develop in parts of the brain that control memory and the retention of learned information. That's why Alzheimer's patients may be very healthy in every other respect. Sometimes the tangles and plaques have also been found in the brains of healthy aging persons who did *not* show any symptoms of a cognitive disorder. These strange ***incongruities*** make it difficult to understand completely how Alzheimer's affects the brain.

Studies have also shown an elevated level of tau in persons suffering from Alzheimer's. Tau is a protein found in the ***cerebrospinal fluid***; a test for high levels of tau may help in a diagnosis of Alzheimer's. Another protein found in the brain is beta-amyloid peptide. While tau levels rise in Alzheimer's patients, beta-amyloid levels fall as senile plaques are formed. These levels can also be tested to help diagnose the disease. Beta-amyloid may cause the ***neurons***

GLOSSARY

incongruities: The appearance of inconsistencies.

cerebrospinal fluid: A liquid secreted from the blood into parts of the brain to maintain a uniform pressure within the brain and spinal cord.

neurons: Grayish or reddish granular cells with specialized processes that are the fundamental functional units of nerve tissue.

Defining Cognitive Disorders, Including Alzheimer's | 19

> As scientists study Alzheimer's, genetic research is adding new links to their growing chain of understanding. Genes located in the nucleus of every cell in the body control the production of enzymes, hormones, growth factors, and proteins. A faulty protein can be produced by slight alterations in the DNA code of a gene. Alzheimer's disease may be linked to problems with the genes on three different chromosomes. Based on this new understanding, researchers have found that a rare form of early-onset Alzheimer's tends to run in families. Scientists are also using genetic information for other studies to further unravel brain disturbances in the later-onset form of the disease as well.

to die; in fact, in one laboratory study, neurons died when beta-amyloid was added to the cell culture. But how or why this happens is still unknown.

AMY plaques are a kind of lesion that was recently discovered in the brain of Alzheimer's patients. These lesions are widespread among people with this disease, just as the other plaques and tangles are. Because of this **prevalence**, AMY plaques are now being studied to determine if they too are a part of the breakdown of neurons in the brain.

A person with Alzheimer's has too much tau, too little beta-amyloid—and both of these may play a significant role in the formation of neurofibrillary tangles and senile plaques. As these abnormal circumstances grow, the normal healthy neurons die—and the patient is less and less able to function.

Although Alzheimer's is the most widespread of the dementias—and one of the leading causes of death in North America—the problems associated with other cognitive disorders are just as devastating. For example, vascular dementia (also called multi-infarct dementia) is perhaps the second most common cognitive disorder. It is caused by a series of small **strokes** within the brain that may or may not be noticed by the patient or those closest to him. As with

GLOSSARY

prevalence: The degree to which something is widely accepted, practiced, or favored.

strokes: Sudden decreased levels of consciousness, sensation, and voluntary motion due to a rupture or obstruction of an artery in the brain.

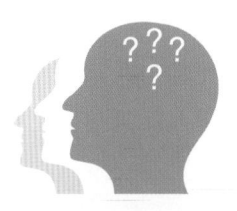

> Many healthy people, including young people, worry about memory loss. Most of this fear is because of the scary reality of Alzheimer's disease. But medical authorities reassure us that very few people under age sixty-four develop Alzheimer's, and only three percent of the population from sixty-four to seventy-four have it.
>
> Still, Alzheimer's is a serious disease. An estimated four million Americans have the disease, and the number is expected to grow to 14 million by the middle of the twenty-first century. The disorder is the third-most expensive disease in the United States (behind heart disease and cancer).

Alzheimer's, brain matter is destroyed, affecting memory and other cognitive functions.

People with Parkinson's disease suffer from a progressive brain disease that causes tremors; slow, shuffling movements; muscular stiffness—and eventually dementia, caused by the depletion of the **neurotransmitter** dopamine. Parkinson's disease is most common in the elderly, but it may be also occur in much younger people; for example, actor Michael J. Fox, who suffers from this disease, has become a spokesperson for Parkinson's. Parkinson's is some-

GLOSSARY

neurotransmitter:
A substance that transmits nerve impulses across synapses.

Causes of Dementia Cognitive Disorders

- Alzheimer's disease
- vascular disease
- other medical conditions, including HIV, head trauma, Parkinson's disease, Huntington's disease, Pick's disease, Creutzfeldt-Jakob disease, substance use

Defining Cognitive Disorders, Including Alzheimer's | 21

times caused by long-term drug use (especially ***antiemetics***), brain trauma or infection, or recurrent strokes. Sometimes its ***etiology*** can't be determined.

Huntington's disease is an inherited, genetic disease. Symptoms commonly begin between the ages of thirty-five and fifty. Children of Huntington's patients have a 50 percent chance of inheriting the gene. The three areas affected by this disease are emotional, cognitive, and motor. Individuals with Huntington's often have involuntary dance-like movements, clumsiness, slurred speech, short-term memory loss, and depression. Although there is no cure for Huntington's, treating the symptoms helps make life more bearable.

Dementia includes many other diseases. Some, like Alzheimer's, Parkinson's, and Huntington's, have no cure, but other dementias can be stopped or reversed. In many cases where cognitive impairment is caused by drugs, depression, thyroid disease, vitamin B_{12} deficiency, ***hypercalcemia,*** and ***hydrocephalus*** (a disease where the brain dies because of lack of flow of spinal fluids), real improvement can occur after medical treatment. Unfortunately, the curable dementias only represent about five percent of the total disease.

A diagnosis of cognitive disorder is often devastating—both for the individual and for the family as a whole. The effects of these disorders are far-reaching. They touch lives at the most intimate levels: socially, intellectually, and emotionally.

> **GLOSSARY**
>
> **antiemetics:** Agents that prevent or relieve nausea or vomiting.
>
> **etiology:** All of the causes of a disease or abnormal condition.
>
> **hypercalcemia:** An excess of calcium in the blood.
>
> **hydrocephalus:** An increase in the amount of cerebrospinal fluid in the cranial cavity, accompanied by an enlargement of the skull and decrease in the size of the brain.

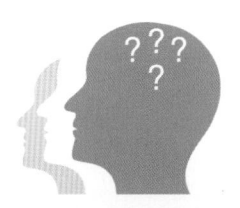

My dear grandchildren,

Sometimes people ask me how I found out I had MCI-Alzheimer's. Because it is a relatively "new" disease, lots of people are interested in learning more about it. Actually, though, it is not a new disease at all—it's just that in the past, the medical community didn't recognize it as a distinct problem. The first symptoms can be rather vague and can mimic many other diseases.

As you probably know, I've had lots of illnesses and surgeries in my life—but usually they had some clear, obvious symptoms that could be checked out and diagnosed. This disease that I have now, however, is very tricky and more difficult to understand. At first, it looked a little like other things I had experienced, whether emotional or physical—but it didn't go away the way those other illnesses did. There was nothing I, or my doctor, could do to make me "better."

Sometimes you probably get tired of my urging you to study hard, and never give up on your dreams. But I want you to achieve all that you want to be, so that you don't feel cheated the way I sometimes do. As you probably know, I fell in love with your grandfather when we were very young, and we married while we were still in college. I got a job and we started our family, but I still always wanted to finish my degree. I took classes one or two at a time until I finally finished a bachelor's degree in social work. Then I went on for my master's degree in counseling. I finally met my goal when I was 50! I first noticed a little trouble with my memory when I was 55, when I went back to school to take some additional graduate courses for my therapist license. For one particular class, there were only two basic exams. I sailed through the first one, which was an essay test, but the second exam required more memorization of facts. I didn't worry too much about it because I'd always done well in school; getting good grades just seemed to come naturally to me. But when I saw the test, I felt absolute panic. My brain seemed to have turned to "mush." I had never experienced anything like this before, and my head and my heart pounded so hard I could barely

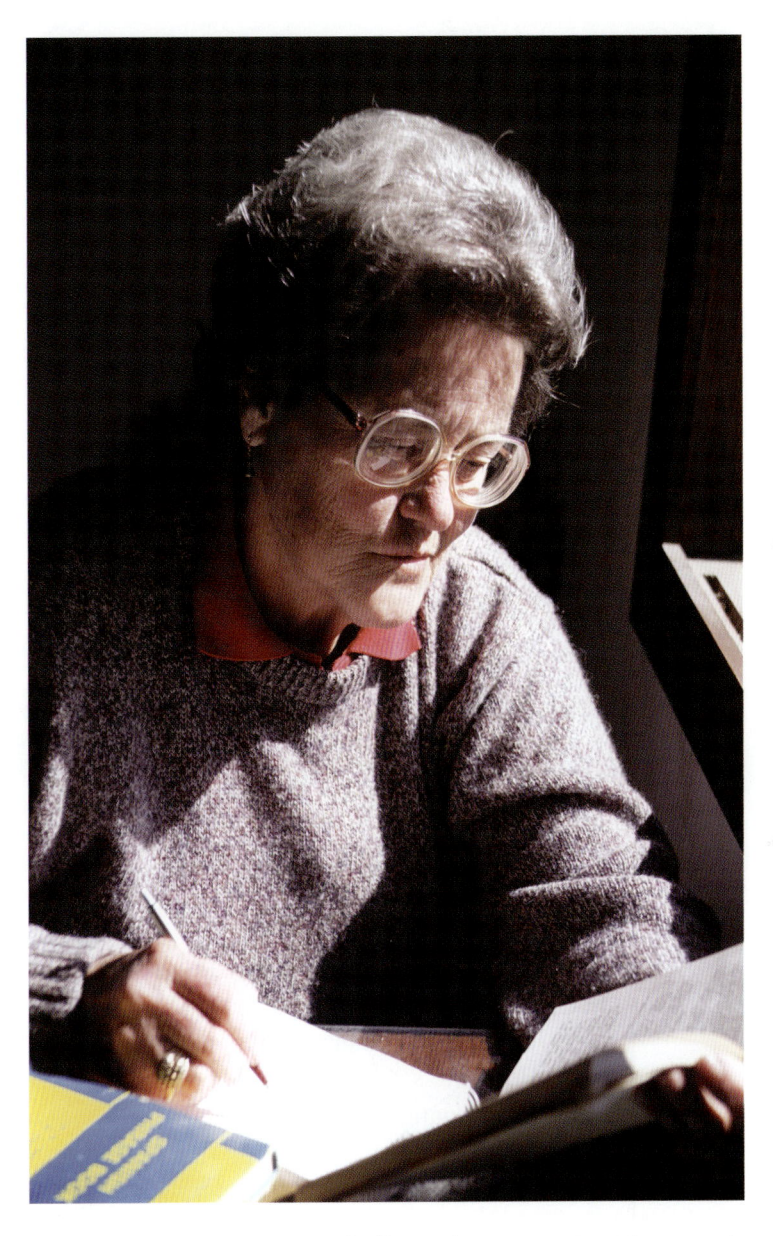

Defining Cognitive Disorders, Including Alzheimer's | 23

Academic work is often a challenge for a person with a cognitive disorder.

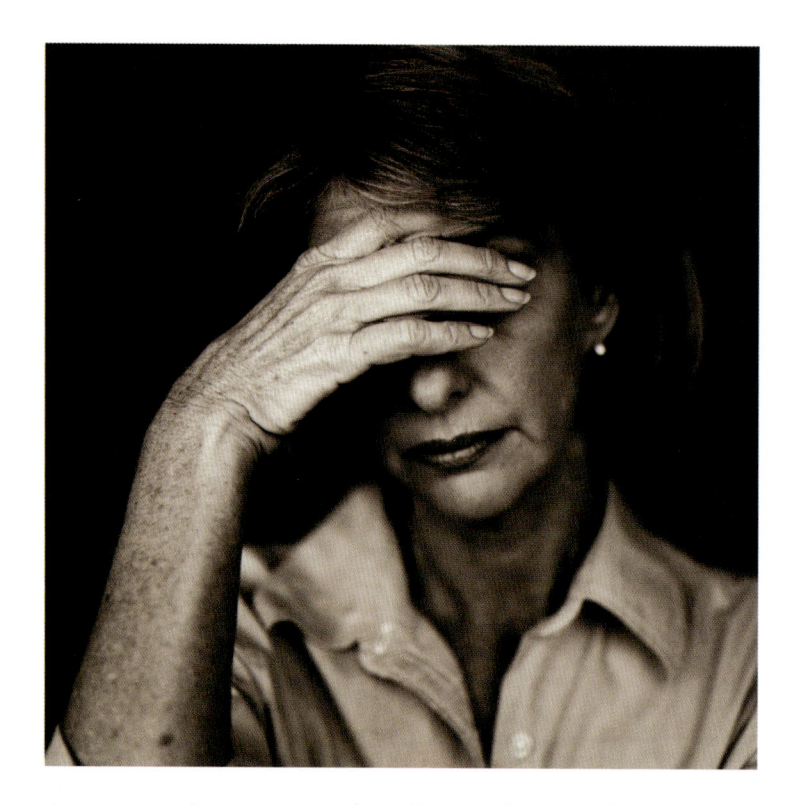

A person with a cognitive disorder may become depressed and anxious.

> On Tuesday, March 13, 2001, the U.S. Food and Drug Administration announced that mild cognitive impairment (MCI) is a condition separate from Alzheimer's disease. Based on this new recognized definition, new drug therapies can be studied to control, stop, or reverse the disorder.

Defining Cognitive Disorders, Including Alzheimer's | 25

> A panic attack is described as a period of intense fear or discomfort in which symptoms develop instantly and reach a peak within ten minutes. Some of the symptoms include palpitations, sweating, trembling or shaking, shortness of breath or a feeling of smothering, chest pain or discomfort, nausea or abdominal distress, dizziness or light-headedness, fear of losing control or going "crazy," and a fear of dying. Panic attacks can be successfully treated with the use of antidepressants and behavior modification.

breathe. This was my first experience with a panic attack; since then, these symptoms have become all too familiar.

I'll write more later, but I need to rest now.

Love,
Nana Carolyn

Loss of memory, personality changes, and the inability to perform normal activities all add stress to the lives of caregivers as well as the Alzheimer's patient herself. On top of all this, the individual may become depressed, anxious, or experience panic attacks like Carolyn does. Other individuals may become aggressive, either verbally or physically. All these emotional symptoms may also make the other symptoms get worse faster. Many people believe this is a part of the disease that must be expected and accepted. But the good news is that in many cases this is not true. Many medications can help control or even alleviate these problems so that the person with a cognitive disorder can live more peacefully. And researchers have also developed medications that can actually improve memory.

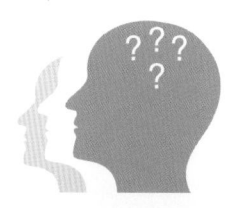

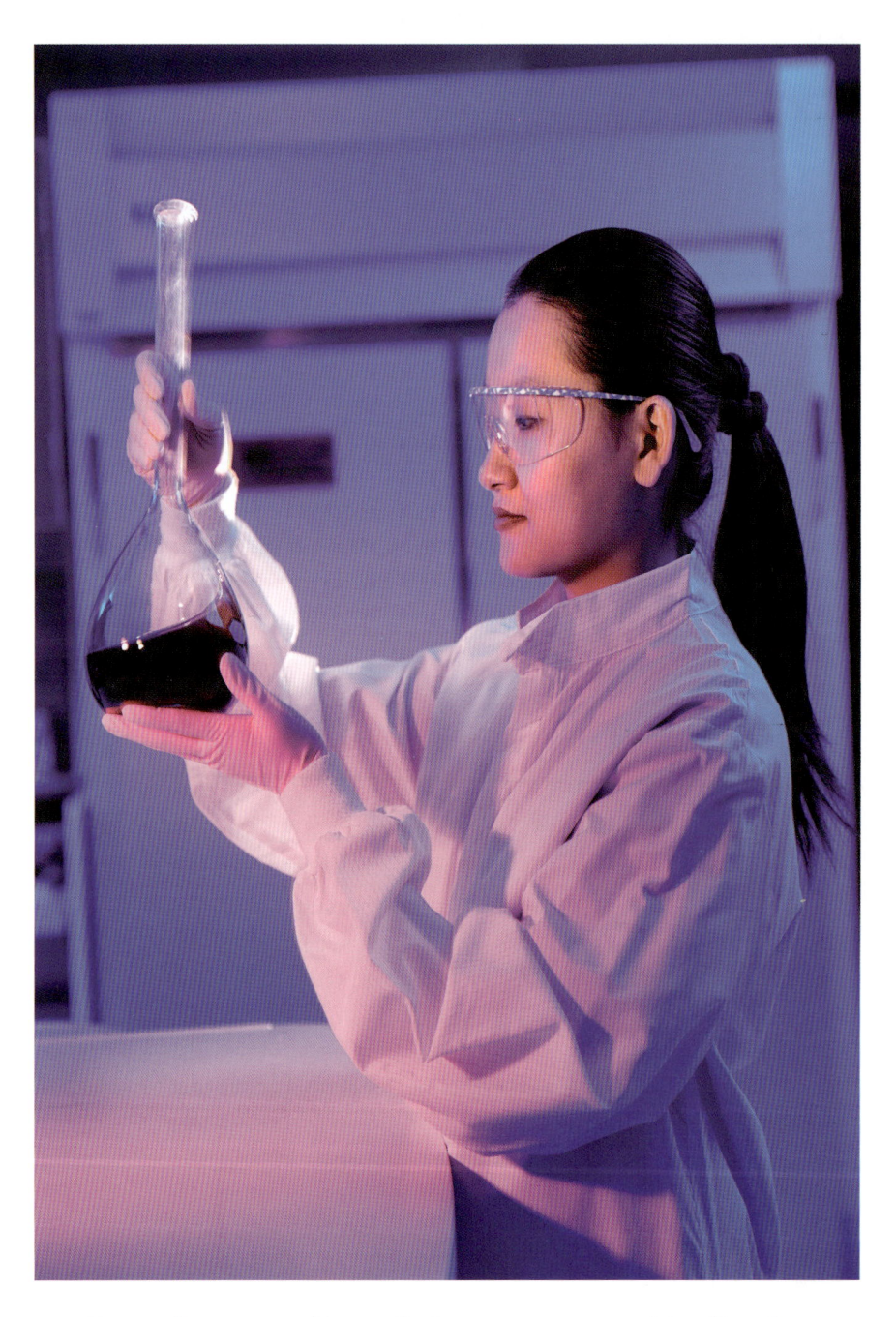

Researchers are working to find ways to treat cognitive disorders.

2 | The History of Drugs' Role in Cognitive Disorders

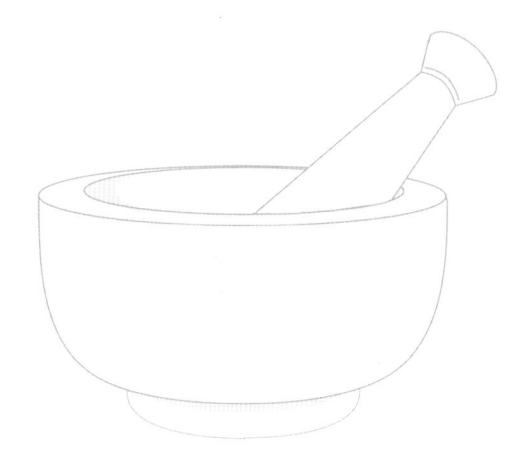

In the 1940s in Australia, Dr. Adrian Albert was looking for a safe intravenous antiseptic to help his nation's war effort in the Second World War. He was intrigued by a drug named tacrine hydrochloride because it had the unique ability to reverse anesthetic-induced sleep.

Later researchers found that tacrine had a broad ability to arouse the CNS from a variety of conditions. In the 1950s, tacrine was used experimentally to reverse certain kinds of coma in animals. By the 1960s, researchers were investigating its ability to reverse the effects of certain drugs, and in 1980, Dr. William Summers demonstrated that tacrine could be used to treat the comas that resulted from certain kinds of drug overdose. Dr. Summers wondered if tacrine might also be used to treat other kinds of brain syndromes—such as memory loss.

Dr. Summers continued his research on tacrine. He demonstrated that the drug did improve (to varying degrees) the memory of those suffering from various stages of dementia. In 1993, tacrine became the first FDA-approved treatment for Alzheimer's disease. A good deal of controversy surrounded the drug, however. Many medical practitioners believed the drug was both ineffective and even dangerous because of the risk of liver damage.

Tacrine was no "magic pill"; it offered no miracle cure to those suffering from a cognitive disorder. But over the years, researchers have searched (and continue to search) for medications that will help people deal with the various symptoms of cognitive disorders.

Some of the most painful of those symptoms are the depression and anxiety that often accompany a cognitive disorder.

My dear grandchildren,

As a counselor I know there are times when a person with a problem or disease gets stuck at a certain place and can't seem to get out. I'm sure you've heard of the word "denial." It happens to a person who finds that facing the truth is just too painful, so she ignores what is happening or hopes it will all just go away. When I first realized something was wrong with my memory, I spent quite a while in denial. I knew something was not right with me but I wouldn't admit it, even to myself. And as long as I avoided correct diagnosis, I couldn't get help.

Remember when Aunt Melissa asked me to come take care of the baby while she recovered from surgery? I loved having the chance to be with some of you—but Aunt Melissa and I both noticed I had trouble remembering her instructions for caring for the baby. I would listen to what she said—but then I'd have to ask her over and over to tell me what to do. After I returned home, she called Grandpa and asked, "What in the world is wrong with my mother?"

The History of Drugs' Role in Cognitive Disorders | 29

"I don't know what you're talking about," Grandpa told her. "There's nothing wrong with your mother. She's the same as she's always been."

That was the first time we heard the word "denial" used for our situation. Aunt Melissa insisted we were deep in denial. Both Grandpa and I were stuck, frozen by our fear. We didn't want to look too closely at what was happening to me, because we were terrified of what we might see.

But I did begin talking to my doctor about my memory problems. He gave me some basic question-and-answer tests and said he didn't see any real problems. Eventually, however, I asked for a referral to a **neurologist**. I was hoping to rule out any possible problems and set my mind at ease.

My first visit at the neurologist's office consisted of answering questions and doing some simple paper-and-pencil tests. Afterward, the doctor assured me I was just having "normal" lapses of memory for anyone with a busy lifestyle. After

> **GLOSSARY**
>
> **neurologist:** A physician who diagnoses and treats disorders of the nervous system.

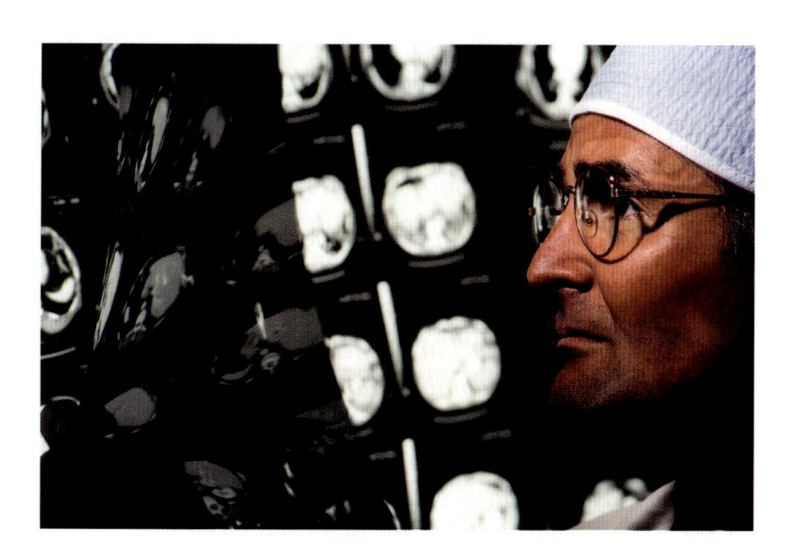

A neurologist may look at brain structures using an MRI.

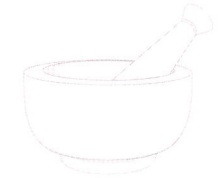

> The brain is very complicated but as with many other parts of the body individuals react differently to treatment. Close observation by a physician is necessary while taking antidepressants to ensure their success. This is especially true with the elderly. Certain antidepressants react with other drugs and, although when used on younger patients they pose no problems, may have more restrictions in those who have weaker hearts, high blood pressure, and other medical problems.

time alone. As they become isolated from their previous lives, their low feelings increase. They may eventually have problems eating and sleeping. All these symptoms of depression can make the cognitive disorder even more severe; their situation may become a vicious circle, where each set of symptoms makes the other set still worse.

That's why an accurate diagnosis is so important for those with cognitive disorders. Once the diagnosis is made, testing for depression will be done on a regular basis. Antidepressants or antianxiety medications may be prescribed to help individuals better cope with their disorder. These drugs help the brain work more efficiently to overcome depression. People like Carolyn may find relief from the depression that had made their memory symptoms worse.

USING DRUGS TO TREAT DEPRESSION

A hundred years ago doctors never considered how depression and cognitive disorders might be interrelated. Memory loss was considered a normal part of the aging process, and old people were often expected to be "crotchety." In the mid-twentieth century, though, researchers began to realize that the brain could be treated with medicine, just like the rest of the body could.

The History of Drugs' Role in Cognitive Disorders

The first antidepressant, iproniazid, was developed in the early 1950s, when physicians who were using the drug to treat tuberculosis noticed that their patients became more energetic and happier—even though their tuberculosis was not improving. These happier patients led researchers to evaluate the drug more carefully to find if it had any effect on those suffering from depression.

Treating depressed patients with iproniazid became common after a 1957 article reported research indicating that the drug improved many of the symptoms of mental illness. The drug was an immediate success from one perspective, but from another perspective, the drug worried physicians. Iproniazid had many side effects, and researchers began to look for another medication that would be safer. Placing their hopes on this soon-to-be-developed, new antidepressant, iproniazid's manufacturer took the drug off the market.

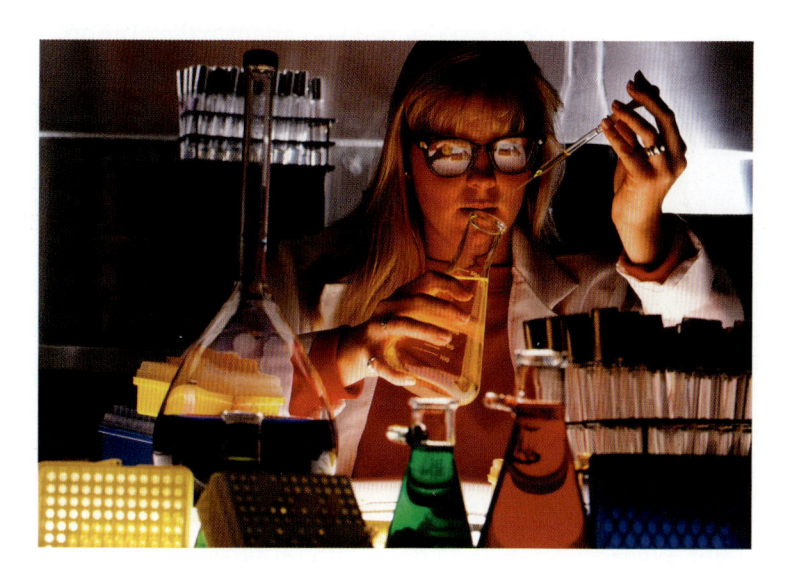

Researchers found that the brain responds to medicine just as the rest of the body does.

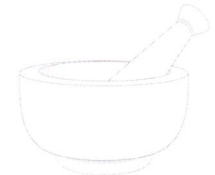

Meanwhile, a leading researcher in Switzerland, Ronald Kuhn, began to look for a specific drug to fight depression that would be nonstimulating in its action so that the person would feel better but not be abnormally energized or agitated. Kuhn began by studying antihistamines, because of the use of the antihistamine chlorpromazine hydrochloride to treat schizophrenia. Chlorpromazine is a *sedative*, so it has a calming effect—but when it was used to treat depression, its success rates were meager. Apparently just calming depressed people did not alleviate their major symptoms.

By the end of 1957, Kuhn announced a substance that would relieve depression. This drug was called imipramine hydrochloride, and it was the first of the antidepressants specifically designed to treat depression without overstimulating the recipient. When people took this drug, their appetites returned, and they became more like their old selves. Most important, they experienced no abnormal elevation of mood; when nondepressed persons took the drug, they simply became sedated. The drug had little chance of becoming addictive.

Imipramine affected the neurotransmitters inside the brain. However, it affected more than one neurotransmitter, so it always caused unnecessary side effects. In effect, parts of the brain were being treated that did not need to be treated—and the more parts of the body altered by a medication, the greater the number of side effects. Imipramine caused the brain to send out messages to the rest of the body as if it were in an emergency situation. People taking the drug felt a little like a person who has just run into a tiger in the jungle: they were ready to either run away or fight. Physicians needed a drug with fewer side effects.

Sometimes researchers create drugs that have the desired effect on the body, but they also have some other effects that are not desired. When this happens, scientists may

> **GLOSSARY**
>
> **sedative:** A chemical that has a calming, soothing effect.

> **Important Information for Treating Elderly Patients with Psychiatric Drugs**
>
> - Diagnosing a psychiatric illness may be complicated.
> - Because the patient may be dealing with other medical problems, there is an additional challenge for treatment choices.
> - The elderly are very sensitive to all medications and may therefore experience more side effects than younger people.

continue their search for a more specific or appropriate drug by creating similar chemicals. They analyze the chemical structure of the drug and then design other drugs with similar structures. Hopefully, these new chemicals will still have the desired effect without the unwanted side effects. This type of research is called homology (from the Greek word *homo*, meaning "same"), because the researchers use the same fundamental structure of the original chemical; they only tinker with the details of the formula. This is often the easiest route where much research begins.

New drugs may also be developed using *analogy*. In this case researchers look for substances that may not look the same chemically but they function similarly. If they have an antidepressant that affects the levels of a particular neurotransmitter in the brain, for example, they look for other substances that will do the same thing.

When imipramine was proven to help depressed patients, researchers used these two techniques to develop other medications similar to it. Some of the antidepressants closely related to imipramine were the monoamine-oxidase inhibitors (MAOIs). Like the first antidepressants, MAOIs

GLOSSARY

analogy: Likeness or similarity between two things that are otherwise different.

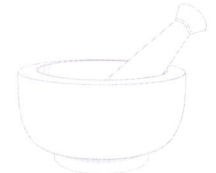

Brand Name vs. Generic Name

Talking about psychiatric drugs can be confusing, because every drug has at least two names: its "generic name" and the "brand name" that the pharmaceutical company uses to market the drug. Generic names come from the drugs' chemical structures, while drug companies use brand names to inspire consumers' recognition and loyalty.

Here are the brand names and generic names for some common psychiatric drugs used to treat cognitive disorders and their symptoms:

Aricept®	donepezil
Exelon®	rivastigmine
Librium®	chlorodiazepoxide
Marplan®	isocarboxazid
Nardil®	phenelzine
Norpramin®	desipramine
Parnate®	tranylcypromine
Paxil®	paroxetine
Prozac®	fluoxetine
Reminyl®	galantine
Tofranil®	imipramine
Valium®	diazepam
Xanax®	alprazolam
Zofran®	ondansetron

worked well when treating depression. Researchers know that this drug **inhibits** monoamine oxidase, a chemical that works in the neurons of the brain, but even fifty years later, scientists still do not understand exactly how these drugs work. Unfortunately, MAOIs can cause hypertension, which meant that for many patients the drug could only be pre-

The History of Drugs' Role in Cognitive Disorders | 37

scribed with much caution. This led to more research for a still better alternative.

Scientists found that imipramine had a chemical structure that looked like three rings, so using the research techniques of homology, they looked at other chemicals with the same three-ring structure. As a result, they developed antidepressants called tricyclics (TCAs).

Many still believed that a particular neurotransmitter, serotonin, held the key to the majority of the mood problems of depression and other diseases. Researchers began searching for a drug that would affect only serotonin within the brain. Finally, in the 1960s, Bryan Molloy, a Scottish chemist, and Ray Fuller, a pharmacologist, worked together at Eli Lilly and Company to find the first drugs that would affect only serotonin—selective serotonin reuptake inhibitors. At the time, Molloy was working on a heart regulator and Fuller was testing new antidepressants on rats. Fuller convinced Molloy to work on chemicals that affect transmitters in the brain, and Molloy began by studying previous work on transmitters. Because much of this research had been based on antihistamines, he decided to start with them, using a model by Robert Rathbun, a third researcher at Lilly. Finally David Wong, a researcher in antibiotics, completed their team when he began studying the role of serotonin in mood regulation.

When Wong learned of the research of Solomon Snyder at Johns Hopkins University, he began using his technology on Molloy's antidepressants. Wong found a way to block the uptake of serotonin without affecting other transmitters. He ran the test on Fuller's rats—and the drug proved to work only on serotonin. Using Wong's studies, Molloy and Klaus Schmiegel, another Lilly researcher, invented a group of synthesized compounds called aryloxphenylpropylamines, which includes the compound called fluoxetine oxalate.

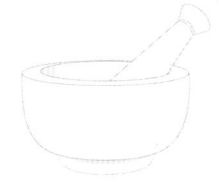

> **GLOSSARY**
>
> ***inhibits:*** *Prevents or discourages something from happening.*

> The selective serotonin reuptake inhibitors (SSRIs) are named after their chemical activity. They inhibit the nerves from reuptaking or reabsorbing all of the serotonin from the synapse after it has been used to send a message between the neurons, thus allowing the brain to retain higher levels of serotonin.

This chemical was then made into fluoxetine hydrochloride—the active ingredient in Prozac.

Prozac was introduced in 1988, about thirty years after the first antidepressants became available. Because of its specific effect on serotonin, Prozac offered relatively few side effects. Patients taking the drug did not feel lethargic or sedated.

Zoloft and the other SSRIs were developed after Prozac. Although these drugs still have some side effects, they are less severe than those of the earlier antidepressants. Finally, drugs had been created that were able to change serotonin levels and affect the brain positively. This meant that people like Carolyn, who suffer from both a cognitive disorder and depression,

Facts About SSRIs

- Since their introduction in 1988, SSRIs have become the most widely used antidepressants.
- Unlike other antidepressants, SSRIs are not addictive.
- Because they change the way the brain works, which can be different for each individual, individual SSRIs do not change one person's symptoms the same way they do someone else's. Sometimes those who take antidepressants must try more than one before they find the one that works best for them.
- At least fourteen subtypes for serotonin exist, which could lead to the development of even more specific drugs that will act on these serotonin subtypes.

could be helped to live more satisfying lives. Although the drug will not make her cognitive disorder disappear, it will help her be able to cope better with the memory loss and other changes that she is experiencing.

USING DRUGS TO TREAT PSYCHOTIC SYMPTOMS

People with cognitive disorders can also benefit from taking other psychiatric drugs. Sometimes people with Alzheimer's and other dementias have trouble sleeping or sitting still. Others have problems with **delusions** and **hallucinations**. They may believe, for example, that people are trying to steal their belongings or injure them in some way, or they may hear voices or see things that aren't real. Symptoms such as these should not be dismissed simply because the person experiencing them is elderly. **Antipsychotic** medications given in very low doses may help people with these symptoms resume a more normal life.

For instance, Frank lived in a nursing home that cared for him well. One afternoon, however, his daughter received a frantic call from him saying that the orderly had stolen his wallet. Concerned, she visited her father that evening. His wallet was in the drawer beside his bed, but when she tried to question him about it, he became agitated and accused her of sneaking poison into his orange juice. Frank's daughter consulted with the nursing home's physician, who arranged for tests to be sure that Frank was not suffering from some other medical problem that might cause his delusions. Then he was given an antipsychotic drug. Within three days, Frank was back to joking with the nurses and orderlies. He was no longer disturbed by the delusion that those around him were trying to hurt him.

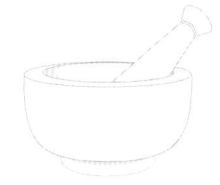

> **GLOSSARY**
>
> **delusions:** False beliefs regarding the self or persons or objects outside the self that persist despite the facts.
>
> **hallucinations:** Sensations that are interpreted by the individual as real, despite the fact that no one else perceives the same things.
>
> **antipsychotic:** Medications that can prevent psychotic symptoms, such as delusions, hallucinations, and impaired reality testing.

> **Facts About Valium**
>
> - Although it has helped millions of people, Valium has been one of the most widely abused prescribed drugs in history.
> - Manufactured by Roche Pharmaceuticals in the early 1960s, the drug was largely unregulated and was often prescribed for problems that did not need the extent of the effect produced on the nervous system.
> - In Mexico and Canada the drug is available in mild doses over the counter.
> - Because of Valium's positive effects, researchers worked to improve on the compound to create antianxiety medications with fewer side effects. Xanax and Dalmane, a hypnotic, are two of the Valium-like drugs with fewer side effects.

USING DRUGS TO TREAT ANXIETY

As Carolyn became increasingly aware of her symptoms, she became more and more anxious. When she was in particular situations where her memory failed her, such as when she was struggling to remember the answers to her exam questions, she was overcome with panic, an overwhelming flood of fear and anxiety. Panic attacks are an all too common experience for many people with a cognitive disorder.

Barbiturates were the first drugs used to treat anxiety during the early 1900s. People who took these drugs experienced feelings of intoxication—much like those caused by alcohol—including slurred speech, impaired judgment, and unsteadiness or lack of coordination. What was worse was the ease with which people became dependent on or addicted to the drug. Overdose was another deadly problem with these drugs, and it became more likely the

> Barbiturates got their name because they were first created by Adolph von Bayer on December 4, 1862—Saint Barbara's Day.

The History of Drugs' Role in Cognitive Disorders | 43

more the drug was used, since dependence tended to lead the patient to use more and more of the drug until he forced his body into a coma or death. Although some people could use barbiturates without these dependency problems, the number who couldn't was high enough that researchers continued to look for alternative medications.

The first benzodiazepines were sold to the public in the 1960s. These drugs were thought to be less addictive and less sedating, but they did not live up to researchers' hopes. When used in higher doses, oversedation, dizziness, and confusion occurred. Again, using the drug often led to addiction, even when it was used at the prescribed doses. However, benzodiazepines did reduce the risk of overdose, since they were not dangerous unless the patient combined them with other drugs or alcohol.

Although these drugs have certain risks, they also have definite benefits, particularly for those who are suffering from a cognitive disorder. Benzodiazepines can help people get more sleep, and these drugs can relieve the worry, anxiety, and agitated feelings that often accompany dementia.

> **Other Drugs Developed to Treat Cognitive Impairment**
>
> - Aricept (donepezil hydrocholoride) was the first drug released to specifically treat Alzheimer's disease. It was launched in April 1997.
> - Exelon (rivastigmine), developed by Novartis Pharmaceuticals, was released in May 1998.

USING DRUGS TO TREAT MEMORY LOSS

At the very end of the twentieth century, researchers announced they had developed a drug designed to improve memory, attention, and decision-making abilities in people

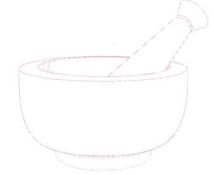

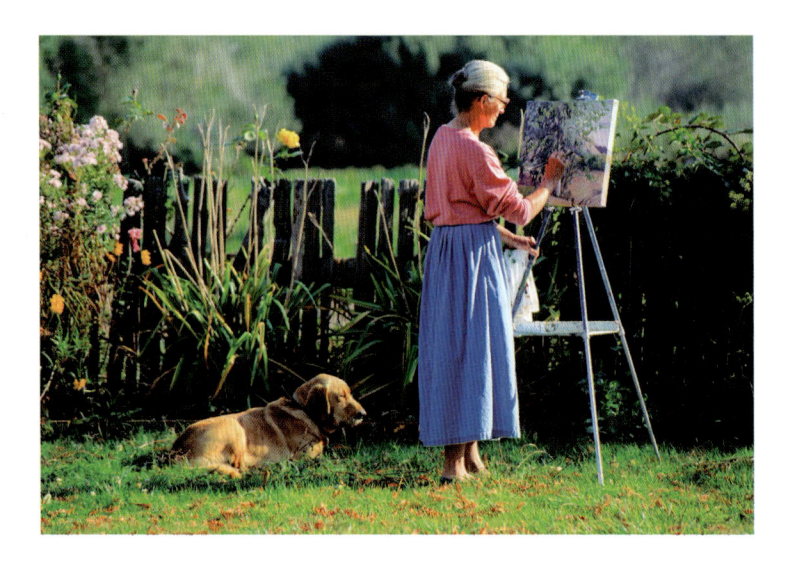

Older people are entitled to lives of creativity and joy.

with Alzheimer's disease. The results of the study were presented in Stockholm in April 2000. The study, by Janssen Research Foundation and Shire Pharmaceuticals, indicated that galantamine hydrobromide helped patients in the early stages of Alzheimer's disease, and those effects lasted for as long as twelve months. These patients had better impulse control, and they could better handle the everyday tasks of life (such as dressing, washing, and feeding themselves). They were also less restless and aggressive, and they experienced fewer delusions and hallucinations. Perhaps best of all, they had better language skills, memory, attention, and decision-making abilities.

Galantamine (with a trade name of Reminyl) was approved for use in the United States in April 2001. It is not the first cognitive enhancer, but it offers the most hope of any developed so far. Research into Alzheimer's is still in its early stages, however, and scientists will continue to look for new and better ways to fight this disease.

As we enter the twenty-first century, the search continues for a drug that will heal human memory. Memory Pharmaceuticals, a biotech firm, is one of the leaders in the race to find effective memory-enhancing drugs. Researchers there use metal electrodes to send tiny jolts of electricity into slices of rat brain. The zap of electricity **simulates** what happens in brain cells whenever a new memory is created in the brain. At the same time, experimental drugs drip into the rat brain cells, while other electrodes measure any changes in the cell activity. Researchers are looking for chemicals that will help the neurons form stronger connections that last longer, therefore improving memory.

> **GLOSSARY**
>
> **simulates:** Copies or represents something else.

SUMMARY

Imagine that a particular nation wants to destroy the evil leaders of another country. The nation's army may attack the other country full force, with powerful bombs. Unfortunately, these bombs will also destroy enormous parts of the entire country, including many innocent civilians. So the warring nation may take another approach—the government may send in assassins that are trained to find and attack only the enemy leaders.

Researchers' war against psychiatric symptoms is a little like that. Scientists continue to seek new drugs to battle depression, anxiety, and other psychiatric symptoms more powerfully—and with fewer side effects. Scientific researchers are hoping to find the "weapons" that will combat the problem, while leaving healthy body functions unharmed.

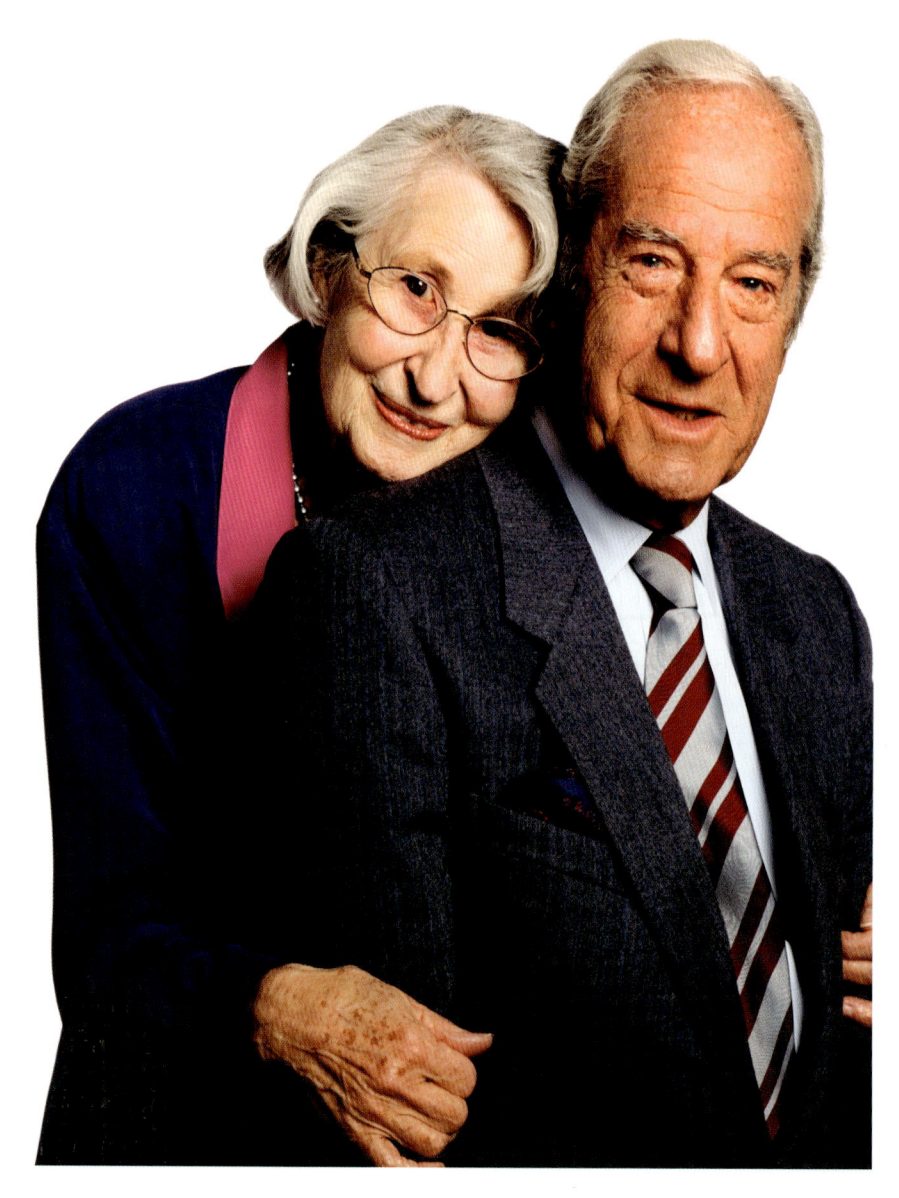

Those who are experiencing a cognitive disorder may be very dependent on their spouses.

3 | How Do the Drugs Work?

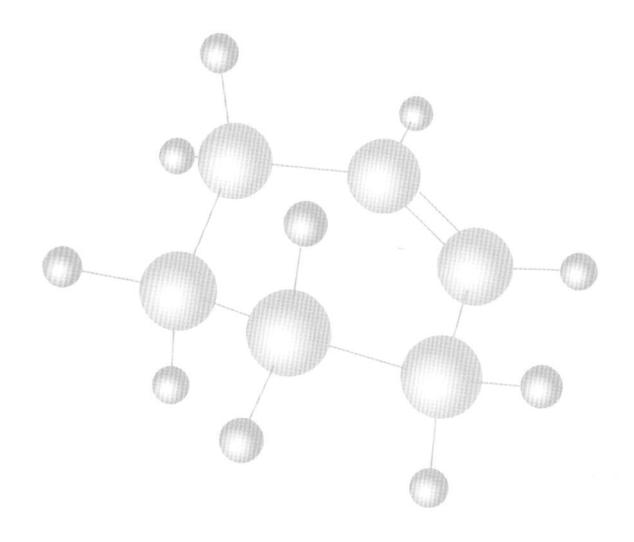

My dear grandchildren,

This disease is hard on Grandpa, too, because he can't do anything to "fix" me or make me better—and that makes him feel frustrated. He is very kind to me, but sometimes my repeated questions about the same thing can make anybody cranky. It is especially hard because up until recently, he counted on me to be the one with a great memory, the one who kept everything organized and running smoothly. For now, I can still keep the house clean and keep up with basic personal care, but for other things I have to rely on him a lot.

For instance, I can't drive myself anywhere because I often forget how to get where I want to go. A few years ago, when we still lived in the city, I drove myself to work every day without a qualm. Now we live in a small, rural community, and I am terrified of getting lost. This is hard for people to understand. It puts an extra burden on Grandpa, and sometimes he gets grouchy.

I still do pretty well with cooking, but I usually cook our favorite dishes, the ones I know by heart. If I cook something new, it's just too frustrating and time consuming—I have to return to the recipe a hundred times because I keep forgetting the ingredients.

It was wonderful being with all of you at Christmas time last year—but it was also stressful for me. People talked to me while I was trying to cook Christmas dinner, which meant I couldn't concentrate on the recipes. People with a cognitive disorder have to stay focused on one task at a time or they can get confused and even more forgetful. And I need to have everything in the same place so I can remember where to find things. After Christmas dinner, your parents tried to help me by putting all my mixing bowls, utensils, and measuring cups neatly away. The first time I tried to cook something in my newly arranged kitchen, I could not find the things I needed. That would seem like a little thing to most people, but for me, because of my disorder, it was enough to trigger a panic attack.

I am learning that many people with Alzheimer's find their memory is worse whenever they are tired, they're in a new place, or they have stressful situations. Those situations take up an awful lot of life, don't they?

Love,
Nana Carolyn

For Carolyn, even life's joys—like a family dinner at Christmastime—can be fraught with stress. Carolyn is still struggling to cope with her emotions on her own, but medication is an option for people like her who may feel overwhelmed at times by their fears, tension, and depression.

If someone such as Carolyn were to take an antidepressant, she would not feel any different most of the time. In other words, the drug does not make a person constantly

NEURONS

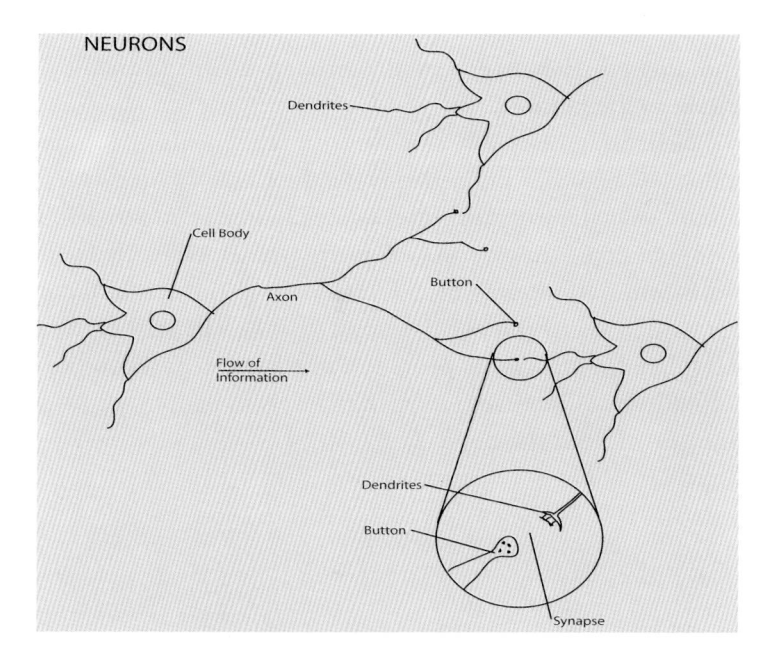

Dendrites
Cell Body
Axon
Button
Flow of Information
Dendrites
Button
Synapse

Neurons pass messages along from cell to cell.

happy. What the drug does do is change the way the body reacts to particular situations. Successful treatment is a quest for alleviating symptoms and allowing the person to function better. Psychiatric drugs can help people like Carolyn feel a little more "normal" again, more like their old selves. For a person who is already struggling with memory loss, release from panic attacks may make living with a cognitive disorder a little easier.

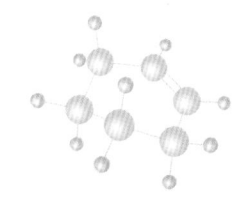

These drugs work within the brain. A healthy brain sends messages throughout the nervous system by way of neurons. The neurons pass along the messages, the way a bucket brigade hands along a bucket of water. The neurons are not connected to each other; in fact, there is a small gap between each one called a synapse. Messages move across the gaps by way of chemicals called neurotransmitters. Once their job of relaying the message is accomplished, they are partially broken down and sent as waste to the kidneys.

Neuroscientists are studying the chemicals that relay messages between the neurons for the cause of Alzheimer's disease. The neurotransmitter acetylcholine is an important component in the process of forming memories. It is the transmitter commonly used by neurons in the cerebral cortex, which is the part of the brain attacked by Alzheimer's. Acetylcholine levels in people with Alzheimer's have been found to be 90 percent lower than levels in people the same age but without the disease.

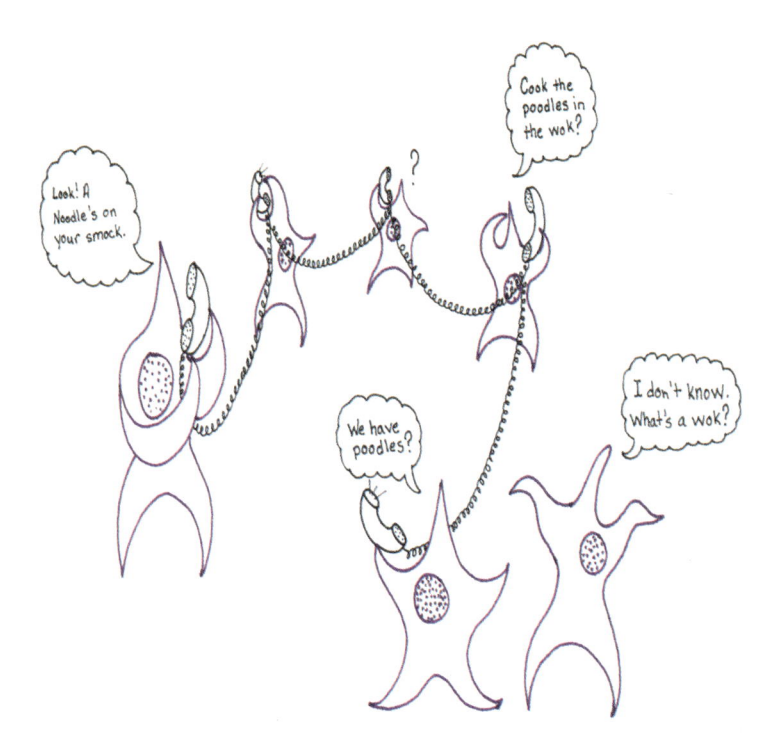

When nerve messages are passed along inside the brain of someone with a cognitive disorder, the message may become garbled—just as the message becomes confused during a game of gossip.

Other neurotransmitters that are affected by the disease are serotonin, somatostatin, and noradrenaline. Levels of all these neurotransmitters are lower in people with Alzheimer's than in healthy persons of the same age. Neuron death may be a result of these lower levels.

In Alzheimer's disease, the molecular bonds within the neuron receptors also show abnormalities. Scientists believe these abnormalities may actually change the messages as they move from neuron to neuron. The shapes of the receptors themselves may affect the messages.

Imagine that you're playing gossip, whispering a message down a long line of people. If someone can't hear very well or can't speak very well, the message is distorted—and what the last person in the line hears may be totally different from the message spoken by the first person in the line. That's a little like what happens in the brains of people with cognitive disorders. The messages passed along by the neurons get mixed up.

After the neurotransmitter has relayed the message in a healthy brain, the remaining transmitters are reabsorbed back into the nerve by a process called reuptake. Each cell that receives a neurotransmitter has thousands of receptors ready to catch it. Imagine a baseball player winding up to throw a ball, with other players standing ready to catch the ball. Now imagine that sometimes the pitcher throws a "ball" shaped like a diamond and other times a "ball" shaped like a square or a circle. Each of the other players has a glove that is designed to catch only a particular shape of ball. The reuptake process is a little like that. Serotonin transmitters can only be received by serotonin receptors, just as norepinephrine transmitters are only received by norepinephrine receptors. By forcing the transmitter to remain in the synapse longer, the brain has more serotonin at its disposal as it sends messages. To accomplish this, reuptake needs to be inhibited to some extent.

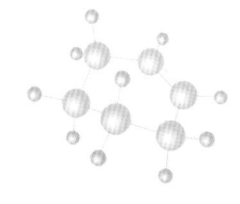

HOW ANTIDEPRESSANTS WORK

Some psychiatric drugs work directly on the reuptake process. TCAs, for example, work by blocking the passage of the serotonin and norepinephrine chemicals from the nerve endings. When this happens, it causes a sedative or tranquilizing effect on the body. They can also elevate mood and help with pain. Tricyclic antidepressants increase mental alertness, physical activity, and can even allow the user to sleep better. When the TCA amitriptyline is combined with the tranquilizer perphenazine, the combination works to treat anxiety and depression.

Serotonin is just one of the transmitters that relay messages within the brain, but it is the one that affects mood and therefore emotion. It is composed of the **amino acid** tryptophan. Serotonin levels help a person to feel calm and relaxed. It also increases control over impulses. Low serotonin levels can make people feel depressed or anxious; they can cause forgetfulness and other symptoms—and yet not everyone who has low levels of serotonin will experience these problems. Apparently, some people are more sensitive to serotonin than others.

Researchers know that persons who suffer from fluctuating serotonin levels experience various symptoms. Because not enough serotonin transmitters are getting to the receptors, the messages are not getting passed from cell to cell as they need to. That's why for the elderly, a problem like dementia can also include depression. The symptoms of being tired, memory loss, and appetite loss can be typical of both dementia and depression. On top of that confusion, someone suffering from dementia may also experience depression simply because he is discouraged

> **GLOSSARY**
>
> **amino acid:** The chief components of proteins that are synthesized by living cells or are obtained as essential components of the diet.

> In monkey societies, the animal with the most serotonin in the brain and nervous system is the highest leader within the community. The most insecure monkeys have the lowest serotonin levels.

How Do the Drugs Work? | 53

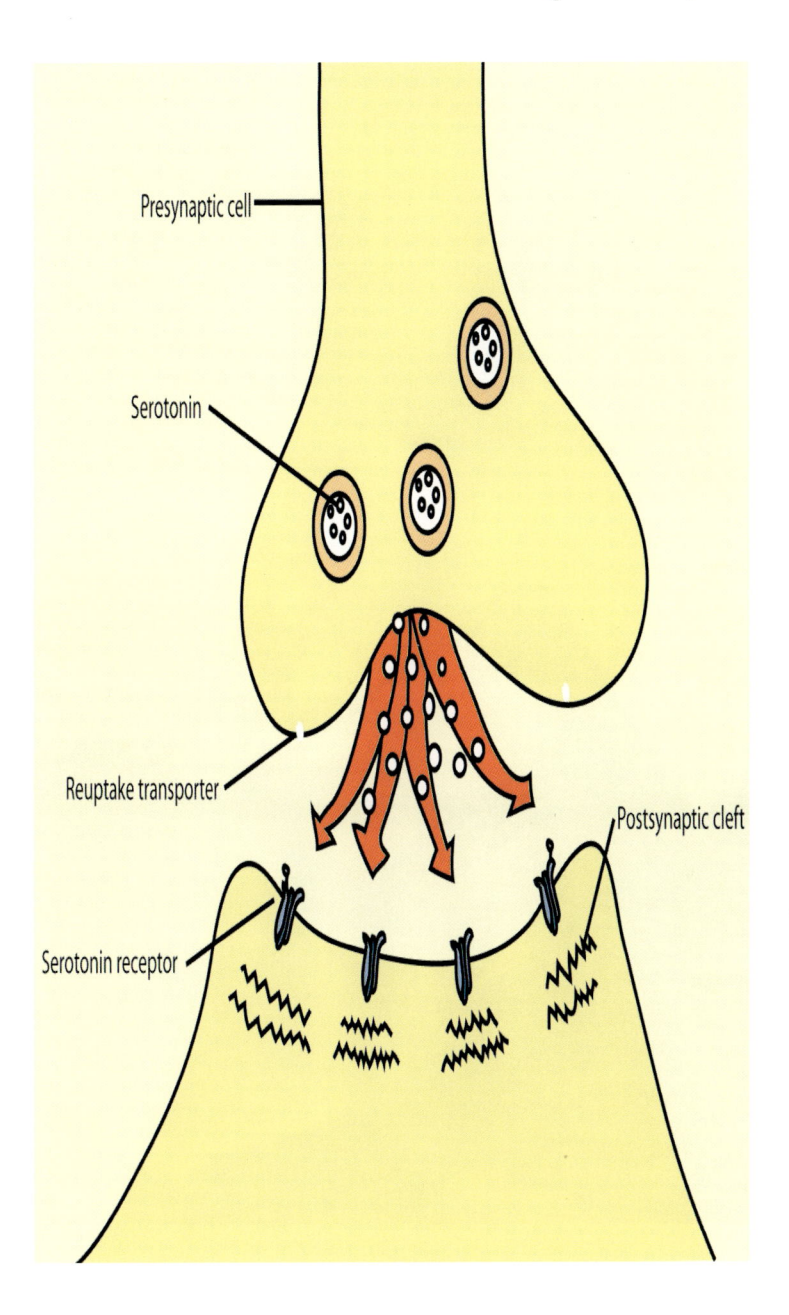

Serotonin helps pass along nerve messages.

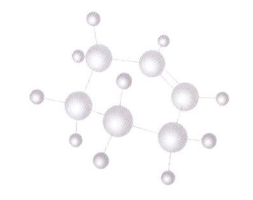

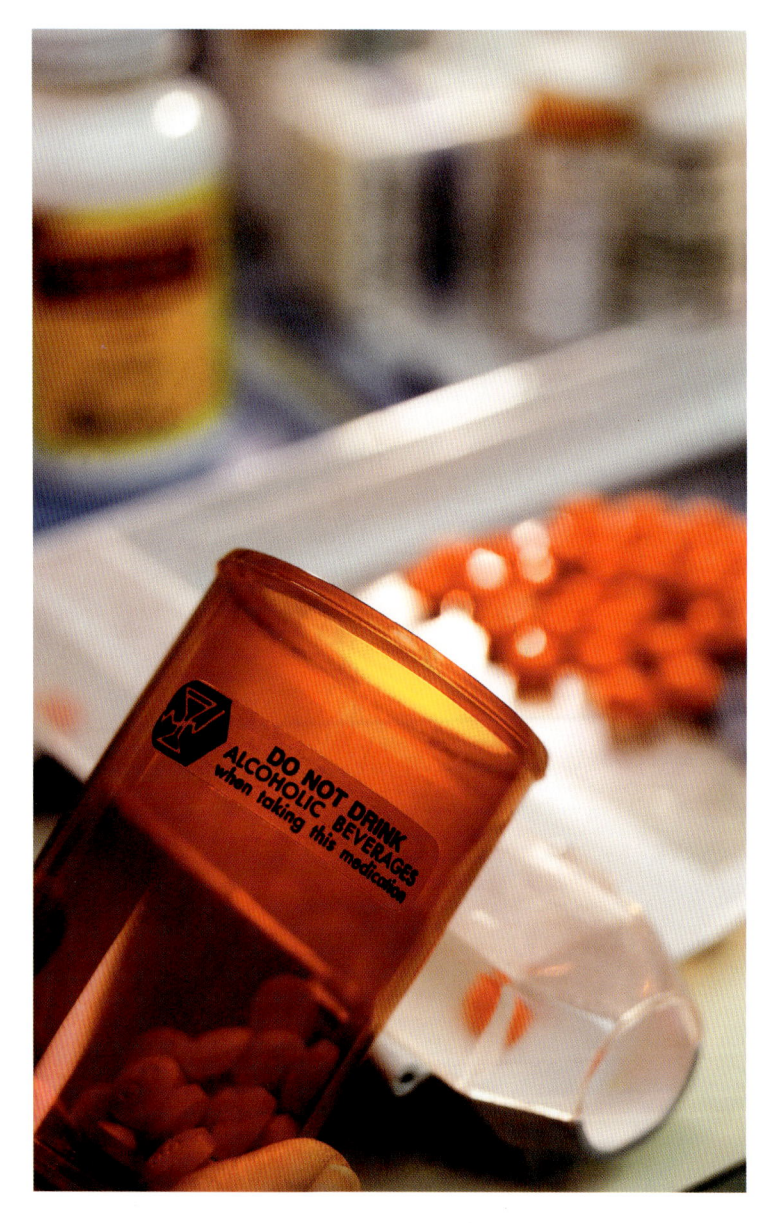

Psychiatric drugs can help a person with a cognitive disorder cope with his symptoms. These drugs are powerful chemicals, though, and they should not be mixed with alcohol or recreational drugs.

and frustrated by his failing mind. Whether the depression or the dementia comes first, antidepressants will lift the patient's mood. And once the person is less discouraged, the symptoms of dementia often improve, even though they cannot be eliminated.

The class of drugs known as SSRIs prevents the neurotransmitter serotonin from moving into the nerve endings. The serotonin is forced to remain in the spaces surrounding nerve endings, allowing the serotonin to act on them. The medication does not produce more serotonin; instead, it is the serotonin *action* that is altered. By making sure that more serotonin is available within the brain, the deficiency is eliminated—and so are many of the symptoms. Antidepressants such as Zoloft and Prozac are SSRIs.

Like the tricyclic antidepressants, the SSRIs also increase mental alertness, physical activity, and allow the user to sleep better, which also affects all aspects of physical and psychological disorders.

As they studied, scientists came to realize the use of serotonin in the brain was very complex. They found that it plays an important role in the brain's control of emotion. They also realized that there is more than one type of serotonin receptor, which may lead to even more specific med-

---

The human brain is an amazing and complex organ, seemingly limitless in capacity. It comprises only about two percent of the body's weight, and yet it coordinates the sensory information experienced by the entire body, allowing the body to react to or process the messages it receives from the outside world. The brain also directs automatic functions in the body, such as the heartbeat and respiration. It releases hormones and controls body temperature and feelings of hunger and pleasure.

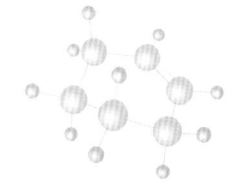

ication that affects just one type of serotonin neurotransmitter.

Unlike tranquilizers that work to slow the body by calming it, Zoloft and Prozac are the regulators. Just like your thermostat in your home keeps the temperature constant, these drugs work to keep serotonin at a productive level within the brain. They accomplish this without making the patient too lethargic and sleepy to perform everyday tasks.

By increasing the levels of serotonin in the brain, researchers have found that confidence and a sense of well-being also increases. Higher levels of serotonin create a greater capacity for concentration, at the same time that it helps a person feel more relaxed. Serotonin also affects how a person feels pain—the more serotonin, the less pain. Also, the more serotonin, the less fear and anger.

HOW ANTIANXIETY DRUGS WORK

Antianxiety medications affect the central nervous system by working in the brain to enhance the functions of GABA, which is the major inhibitor of nerve transmission between the brain and the CNS. You might say it acts to slow down the nerve messages.

One of the benefits of antianxiety medications such as benzodiazepines is that they are very fast acting, so the patient experiences relief almost immediately. Because of this, they work well in emergencies or for short-term therapy. However, those taking these drugs must be monitored closely because of their addictive qualities. They are typically used short term to decrease anxiety while the person is waiting for an SSRI to become effective. Once the SSRI is working, the person may only need to take a benzodiazepine once in a while for "break-through" anxiety. However, if the patient finds she needs to take a benzodiazepine

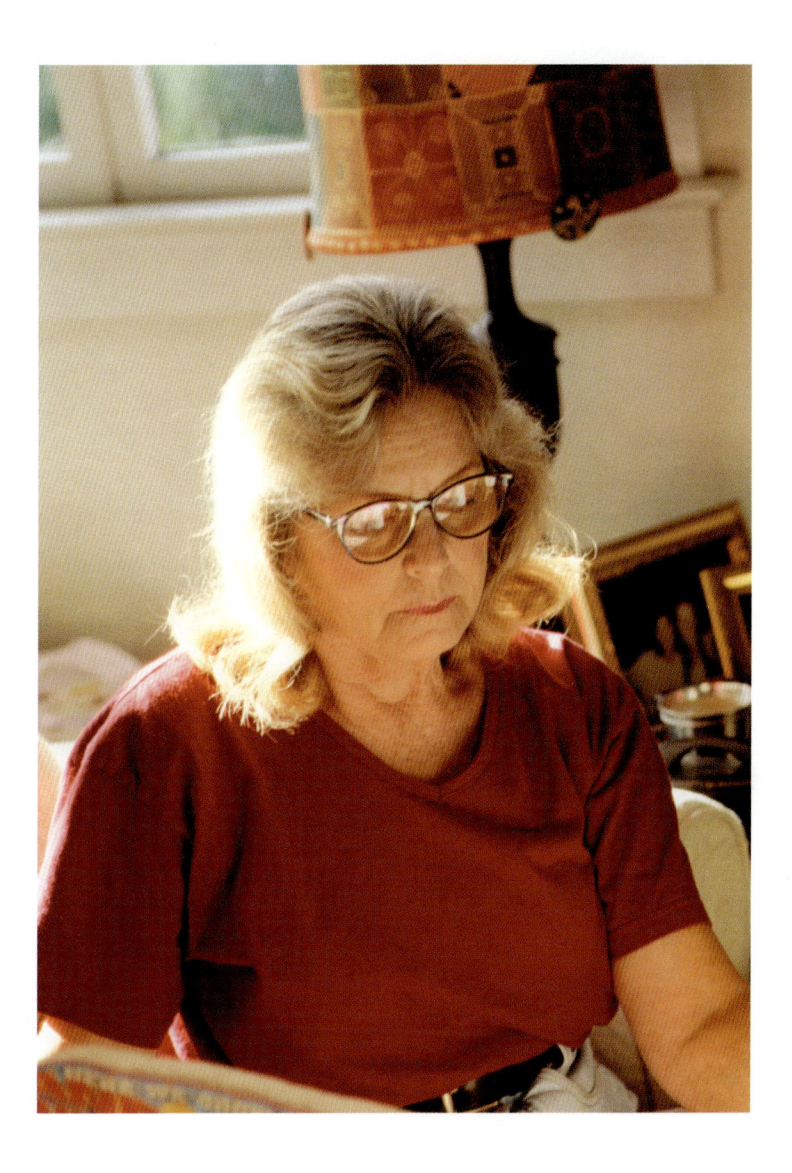

Higher levels of serotonin can help people with a cognitive disorder achieve greater mental focus.

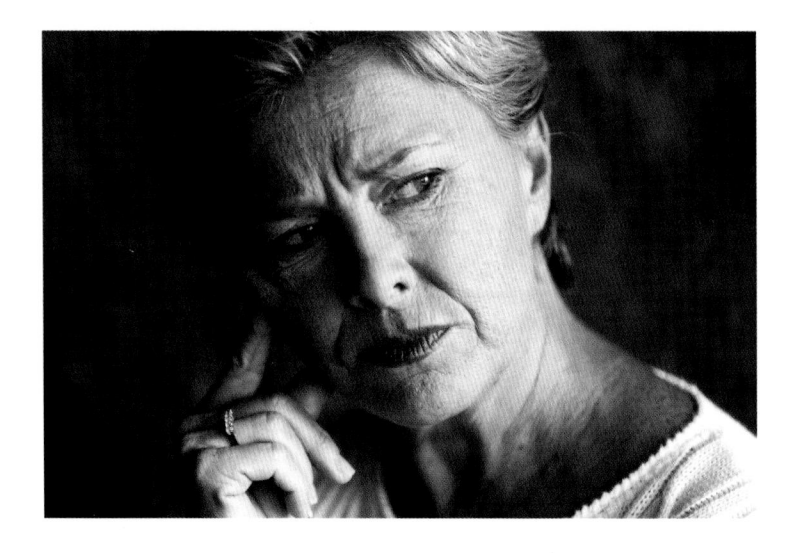

A person with a cognitive disorder may become preoccupied with worries as she struggles to remember schedules and other details of life.

in addition to her SSRI more than once a week, she should notify her medical practitioner, since this may be a sign that the SSRI needs to be increased or changed.

Tranquilizers are taken orally, and once in the bloodstream they are moved to the liver where they are **metabolized**. From the liver, the useable parts of the drug attach to proteins in the blood and are transported to the brain. There, they begin to affect the normal functioning of the brain by repressing neuron activity or holding it back. In the thalamus, where much of the receiving and transmitting of messages occurs, things like pleasure, pain, and hot or cold are affected. By sending messages to the hypothalamus, where emotions such as anxiety, fear, and anger are felt, the drug is able to regulate the messages then sent to the rest of the body.

When a person is taking a tranquilizer, feelings of fear are lessened; people no longer experience the overwhelming

---

GLOSSARY

metabolized: *Changed the chemical composition in living cells by which energy is provided for vital processes and activities and new material is assimilated.*

sense of impending doom that is so often felt during an anxiety attack. Tranquilizers are ideal for a patient who is suffering while becoming accustomed to some change in his life. The short-term use of the medication makes it much more effective and less addictive.

For people with cognitive disorders, anxiety may often be a problem, as it is for Carolyn. They may seem jumpy, irritable, or scared most of the time. For example, when Alma came to live with her daughter Francine and her family, Alma was suffering from the beginning stages of Alzheimer's disease. She could still function well on her own, but she was forgetting phone numbers and doctor's appointments. Francine felt that if her mother stayed with them she could continue her own life but have the help of family members to monitor the things she might forget. Things were fine for the first week, but soon Alma began worrying so much that she could not sleep.

Alma couldn't seem to understand the grandchildren's school schedules. She worried about where they were throughout the day, and she wondered where Francine went when she volunteered at a local clinic two afternoons a week. Soon Alma was so preoccupied with her worries that she no longer cared for herself as well. Every little noise made her jump.

Francine took her to her physician. He gave Alma some tests that all came back negative. After questioning both mother and daughter, the doctor diagnosed Alma with anxiety. He said that anxiety was a perfectly normal reaction to any major changes in life. After all, even though Alma wanted to make the move to Francine's, she was also concerned that she would be a burden to her family. She had lived alone for a long time, and the noise and busyness of her daughter's house was hard for her to get used to. Her memory loss, caused by Alzheimer's, just made her worries that much harder for her to handle.

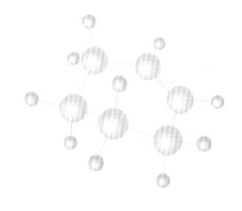

> Alzheimer's disease often occurs in stages. Doctors may use the Functional Assessment Staging Scale to assess a patient.
>
> - Normal adult who has no functional decline.
> - Normal older adult who recognizes he has some functional decline.
> - Early Alzheimer's patient notices problems in demanding situations.
> - Mild Alzheimer's patient who requires assistance in completing more complicated tasks such as finances and travel.
> - Moderate Alzheimer's patient who requires assistance in choosing the appropriate clothing to wear each day.
> - Moderately severe Alzheimer's patient who requires assistance dressing and bathing and may become incontinent.
> - Severe Alzheimer's patient who is unable to speak except for a few words. Eventually loses the ability to walk, sit up, smile, and hold up his head.
>
> Adapted from Barry Reisberg, M.D.

Her physician prescribed a low dose of an antianxiety medication. He also recommended that Alma be moved to a back bedroom where she would have more quiet. He advised the family to try to keep things as calm as possible until Alma had adjusted to her new surroundings.

HOW COGNITIVE ENHANCERS WORK

Reminyl, Cognex, Aricept, and Exelon are all cognitive enhancers designed to improve memory, attention, and decision-making abilities in people in the early stages of Alzheimer's disease. These drugs all belong to the class of drugs known as acetylcholinesterase *inhibitors*.

Research has shown that people with Alzheimer's don't have enough acetylcholine in their brains. As discussed

GLOSSARY

inhibitors: Things that get in the way of an action.

before, acetylcholine is a neurotransmitter, and without it, the human brain does not work properly, creating the symptoms of Alzheimer's. Drugs such as Reminyl inhibit acetylcholinesterase, the **enzyme** that breaks down this neurotransmitter. As a result, these drugs produce higher concentrations of the missing neurotransmitter, leading to increased communication between the nerve cells. This temporarily improves or stabilizes Alzheimer symptoms.

Reminyl, Aricept, and Exelon also appear to stimulate the nicotinic receptors to release more acetylcholine. Nicotinic receptors are located in the brain, spinal cord, and muscles. Researchers believe that these receptors are involved in **cognition**, pain, and **neurodegeneration**. Stimulating these receptors to release more neurotransmitters

> **GLOSSARY**
>
> **enzyme:** A complex protein produced by living cells that causes specific biochemical reactions at body temperature.
>
> **cognition:** The act or process of knowing.
>
> **neurodegeneration:** The deterioration of nerve tissue.

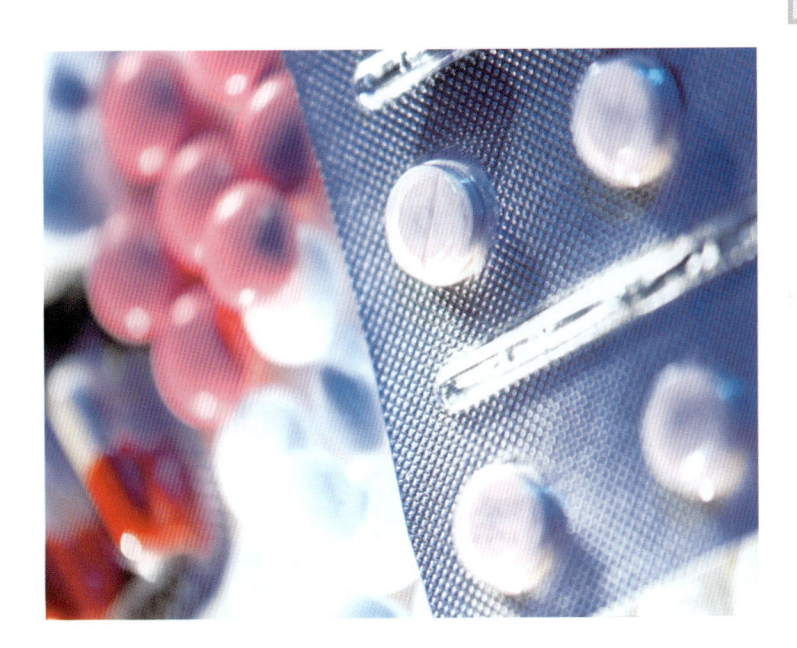

Medication offers new hope to those with memory loss.

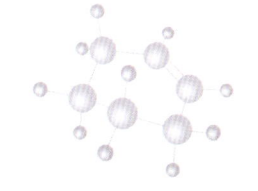

62 | CHAPTER 3

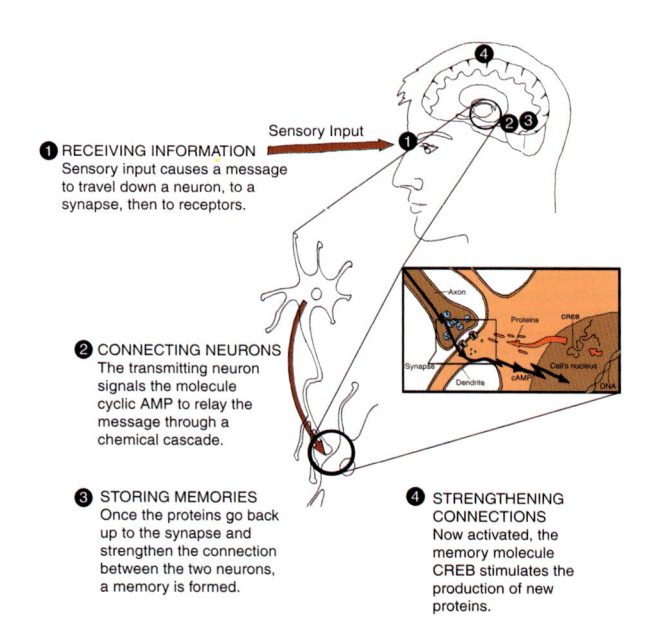

① RECEIVING INFORMATION
Sensory input causes a message to travel down a neuron, to a synapse, then to receptors.

Sensory Input

② CONNECTING NEURONS
The transmitting neuron signals the molecule cyclic AMP to relay the message through a chemical cascade.

③ STORING MEMORIES
Once the proteins go back up to the synapse and strengthen the connection between the two neurons, a memory is formed.

④ STRENGTHENING CONNECTIONS
Now activated, the memory molecule CREB stimulates the production of new proteins.

This diagram illustrates how memories are formed inside the brain.

helps to improve Alzheimer's symptoms as well as the symptoms of Parkinson's disease and schizophrenia.

Tacrine (Cognex) has numerous mechanisms of action. Like Reminyl and Aricept, it is an acetylcholinesterase inhibitor, but it also blocks sodium and potassium channels and alters the uptake of serotonin and noradrenaline. It also increases the release of noradrenaline and dopamine, and stimulates cholinergic firing—all of which have been proven to be related to the symptoms of cognitive dysfunction. Alzheimer's disease is also associated with decreased blood flow in the brain, and tacrine significantly increases cerebral blood flow in patients who have Alzheimer's disease. It also blocks the secretion of the protein that creates the amyloid deposits in the brain. Because of its wide range of action, some researchers believe that tacrine is uniquely suited to treat Alzheimer's disease. However, other researchers fear that tacrine's side effects are too dangerous to justify its use. This medication is somewhat controversial, and as a result, it is not prescribed as often as the other cognitive enhancers.

SUMMARY

People like Carolyn who suffer from the early stages of a cognitive disorder may feel anxious and embarrassed about their symptoms. They may feel guilty that they are causing their family so much difficulty, while friends and family members may feel frustration and even anger at the memory loss the person is experiencing.

A cognitive disorder is caused by things beyond anyone's control. When things go wrong inside the brain, there is never a simple way to "fix" the problem. Cognitive enhancers and psychiatric drugs, however, have the power to change the way the brain works. They cannot make the problem disappear, but they can reduce its symptoms.

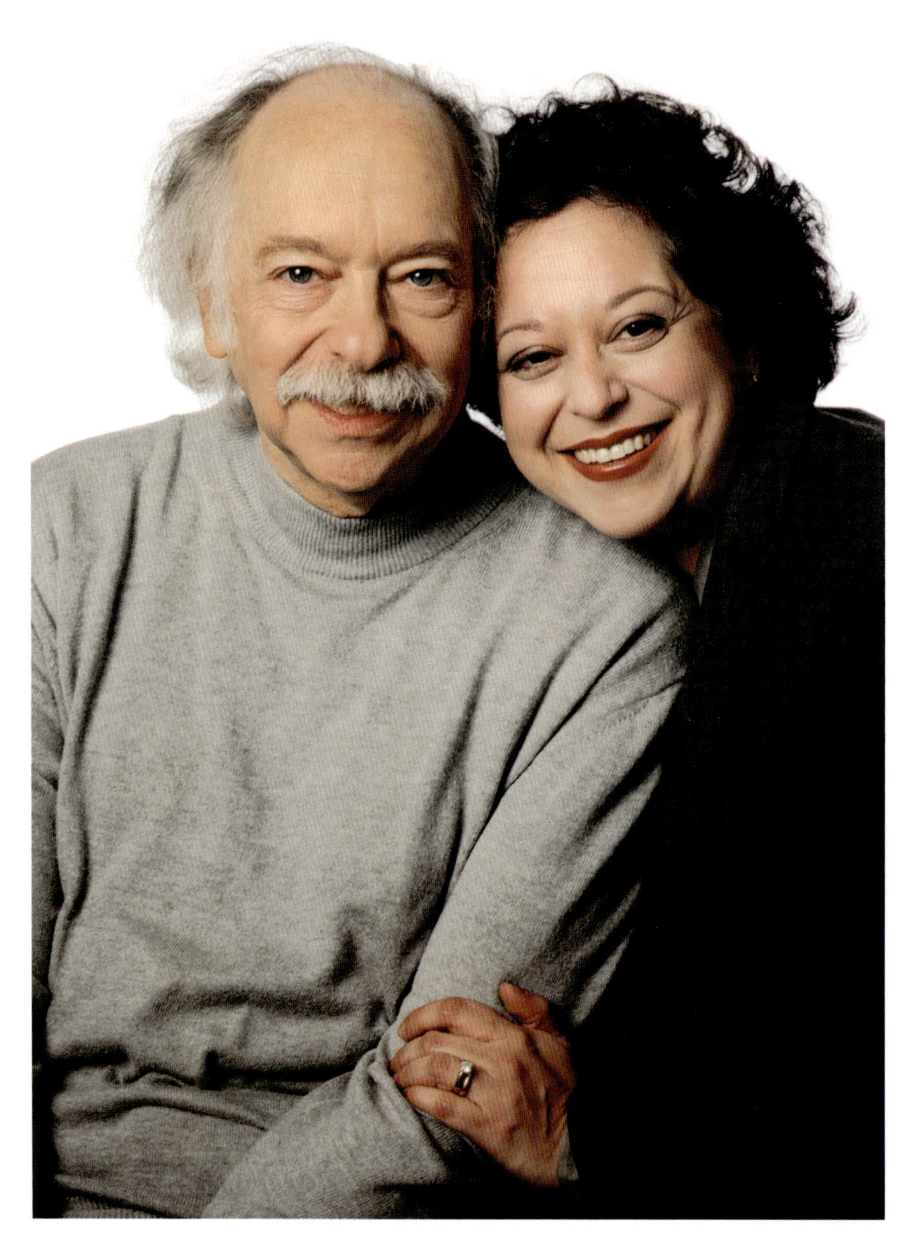

People who experience a cognitive disorder need plenty of love and support from spouses, friends, and other loved ones.

4 | Treatment Description

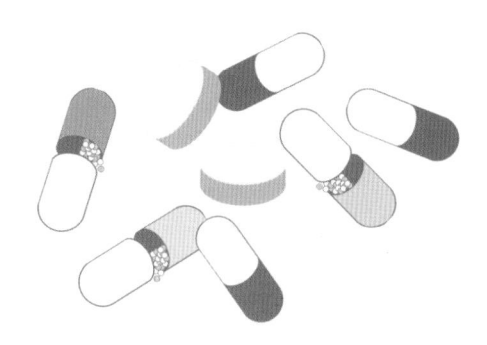

My dear grandchildren,

I was really scared the first time I went to the large teaching hospital at the university campus. The university was performing a special study on people who were diagnosed by their physicians with short-term memory problems, including MCI. The research was to confirm whether or not there is a stage of memory loss before the diagnosis of Alzheimer's disease. Even though they had all their test participants selected, the researchers had agreed to see me anyway. As Grandpa drove through the rush-hour traffic, all I could think about was how scared I was to go to this huge teaching hospital and talk to a bunch of strangers about my memory problems.

We finally found the reception area for the clinic and were asked to fill out a bunch of forms that seemed to take forever. Worst of all, the receptionist insisted that Grandpa had to fill them out even though the information was mostly about me and how I feel and act. I wondered, If this is about me, why don't they ask me? *I felt as though I were no longer the competent, professional person I had once considered myself to be; instead, I felt like someone second-rate and inadequate, someone who could no longer speak for herself.*

We spent the whole day there because they gave me a lot of tests. Most of these tests were timed, and I had to remember and say things as quickly as I could. For example, I had to name as many animals beginning with the letter "G" as I could or count using different sets of numbers. Some questions were about current events.

After all the different tests were reviewed, the group recommended that I be included in the study, even though it had already started. The researchers were going to try a different medication and see if it was helpful to people with my condition. The goal is to see if anything can stop mild cognitive impairment from progressing to Alzheimer's disease.

I'm almost afraid to hope.

Love,
Nana Carolyn

Researchers are constantly looking for medications to fight the many diseases that attack human beings. Alzheimer's and other cognitive disorders are some of the most mysterious of all human diseases. Research for medication to tackle these disorders is only just beginning. In the meantime, the psychiatric symptoms that accompany cognitive disorders are often addressed with drug therapy.

Treating people with cognitive disorders with any drugs, but especially psychiatric ones, requires much effort by the physician, the patient, and often a caretaker. All physical problems must be monitored. Even over-the-counter drugs must be considered for possible side effects. Some physicians are so afraid of the possible side effects that they do

Treatment Description | 67

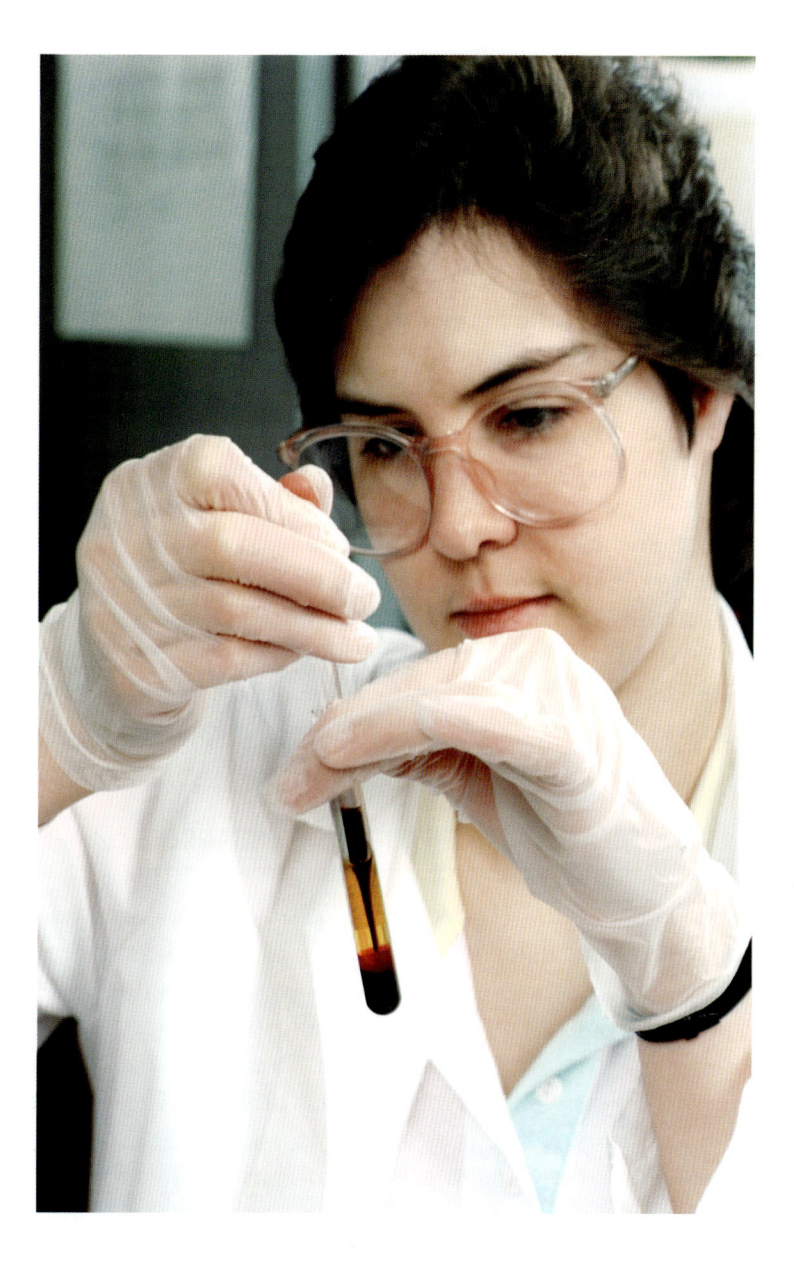

Researchers are constantly seeking new answers to the diseases that trouble humanity.

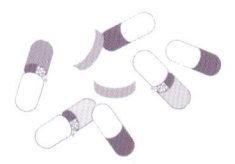

not treat psychiatric illness in patients with cognitive disorders, particularly if those patients are elderly.

Many doctors, however, are now convinced that quality of life does not need to be abandoned simply because a person has a cognitive disorder. After a physical and mental evaluation of the patient, these physicians will often prescribe either an antianxiety medication, an antidepressant, or in some cases an antipsychotic.

Being sure of the diagnosis is the first step to accurate treatment. Sometimes this is more difficult because of complications from other diseases. Many people with cognitive disorders are elderly—which means that they are also more like to have another medical condition. The chance of an underlying medical problem must be ruled out, since a large number of medical problems—such as cancer, hormone disturbances, heart problems, and unrecognized strokes—can also cause psychiatric symptoms. Once a person has been diagnosed with a cognitive disorder, it is important to choose the right drugs to treat the various symptoms.

TREATMENT WITH COGNITIVE ENHANCERS

No one can definitely predict the results of any drugs designed to treat dementia. Some people who take the drug will improve, others will find that their condition becomes stabilized, but still others will continue to get worse.

Reminyl is available in tablets. One 4-, 8-, or 12-milligram tablet is taken twice a day with food. The recommended starting dose is 8 milligrams a day for at least four weeks. After that time, the physician may reassess the dosage.

Donepezil (Aricept) comes in tablet form to be taken usually once a day in the evening just before going to sleep. Donepezil may be taken with or without food.

> **What kinds of questions should a person ask her doctor before taking Reminyl?**
>
> - What benefits can I expect from taking Reminyl?
> - How long will it be before I see a result?
> - How might the drug affect my other medical conditions?
> - What other drugs might interact with Reminyl?
> - How does Reminyl compare to other cognitive enhancers such as Aricept and Exelon?
> - If I am already taking Aricept or Exelon, should I switch to Reminyl?
>
> Adapted from the Alzheimer's Society Web site.

Rivastigmine (Exelon) comes as a capsule and is usually taken twice a day with meals. Patients generally start on a low dose of rivastigmine and gradually increase the dose (not more than once every two weeks). If someone experiences severe stomach side effects, such as upset stomach and vomiting, he may need to stop taking rivastigmine for a few doses and then start taking it again at the same or lower dosage. If a person stops taking the drug for more than a few days, he should talk to his doctor before starting to take it again. (He will probably have to restart taking it at the lowest dose.)

Tacrine is rapidly absorbed. Taking it with meals can reduce absorption as much as 40 percent. Since each person responds very differently to tacrine, it is essential to personalize the dose. The initial dose is 10 milligrams four times each day. After four weeks, if the patient is tolerating the drug, the dose can be increased to 20 milligrams four times a day.

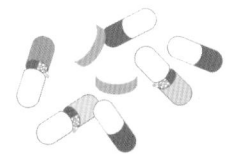

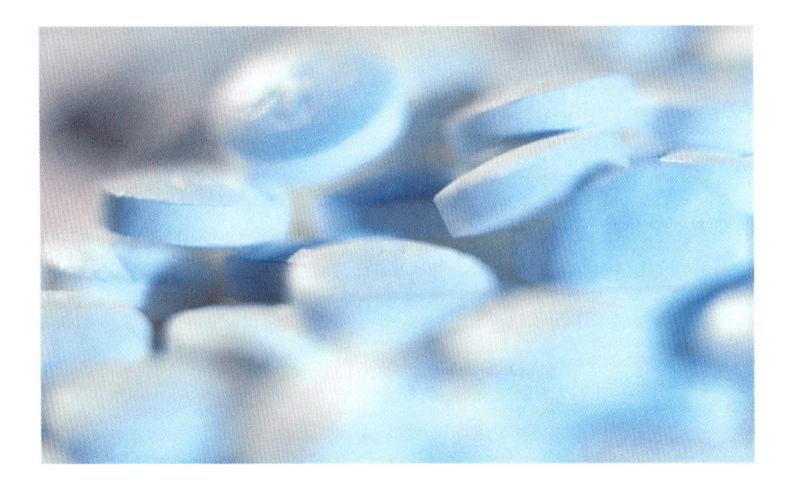

No one should ever take more of a medication than what has been prescribed.

All of these drugs should be taken exactly as directed. Sometimes people think, *If a little of this drug will help my memory a little, a lot of the drug will help my memory more.* But the body's response to these chemicals is never that simple. People should never take more or less of any medicine than what was prescribed by their practioners.

TREATMENT WITH ANTIDEPRESSANTS

Prozac is an SSRI antidepressant that can be started with a 20-milligram dose but should not exceed 80 milligrams per day. Elderly patients are better off if they start at about half the dose of a younger person. For those who have trouble with anxious feelings, one pill can be taken every other day. The medication remains in the body for several days after discontinuing the drug and has been found in the blood weeks after terminating use—which means a person more sensitive to the drug can get the same benefits on an every-other-day dose.

When treating depression, some patients may improve within two weeks, but most will take up to six weeks to feel improvement. Those who have trouble sleeping while taking Prozac should take their medication in the morning. This is sometimes the only adjustment needed to alleviate this problem.

One of the most important precautions to remember about taking **SSRIs** is that there can be a very dangerous, or even fatal, reaction between one or the other of these drugs and the monoamine oxidase inhibitors (MAOIs). If the patient is presently taking any of the MAOIs, drugs—such as Nardil, Parnate, Marplan—or has quit taking one within the past two weeks, he should not begin taking Zoloft or Prozac without consulting his physician.

Zoloft is another of the **SSRIs** approved for depression and panic. The usual starting dosage for adults is 50 milligrams once a day, either in the morning or the evening. For those having a problem with insomnia, Zoloft should be taken in the morning. Zoloft is available in 25-milligram, 50-milligram, and 100-milligram scored tablets, which can be divided to allow adjustment of dosages. Those who are sensitive to medications, like the elderly, should start out at 25 milligrams, which can then be increased after a week or more of treatment but should not exceed 200 milligrams per day. A dose may be crushed and mixed with food or left in tablet form. There is no problem taking Zoloft without food, but food does enhance absorption.

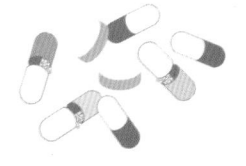

Like Prozac, patients usually need four weeks to feel the full effect of Zoloft, but some need as long as eight weeks. If a dose of Zoloft is missed, it must be taken as soon as possible. If several hours have passed, however, the dose should be skipped, as no one should ever take a double dose. The pills are best stored at room temperature. As with Prozac, the physician should always be informed of any changes that occur—good or bad—while taking Zoloft.

There have been many trials done studying the effectiveness and safety of Prozac and Zoloft. These drugs are considered safe to use but must be monitored by a doctor regularly because each person reacts to medication differently. Some people are so sensitive they need to adjust their dosages and to start at very low levels, moving slowly up to the lowest effective dose.

For patients with cognitive disorders, stress can make their memory problems worse. Some physicians prescribe a low dose of an antidepressant such as Prozac to help the brain function more efficiently. Physicians have found that anxiety, panic, and mood swings can lead to increased forgetfulness. Therefore, a low dosage of an antidepressant can

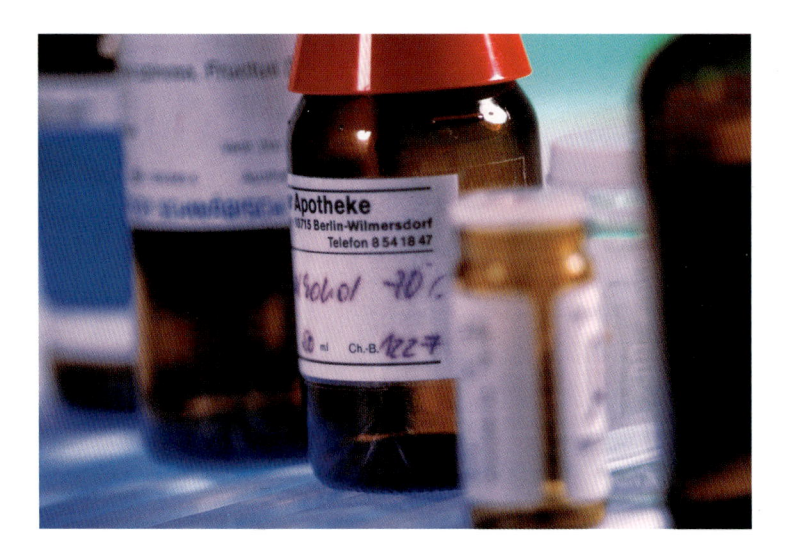

Whenever a person is taking a medication, she should be evaluated frequently by a medical practitioner.

> ## "Off-Label" Prescriptions
>
> The FDA bases its approval on specific research results. Sometimes, a particular use for a drug may have been thoroughly researched by many studies, while other uses lack the same amount of research. In that case, the drug label will only include the uses that have met the FDA's stringent research requirements. Physicians, however, may continue to prescribe that drug for other "off-label" uses.

often help control the immediate symptoms of a cognitive disorder before they lead to a larger problem.

One of the most commonly used TCAs in the treatment of people with cognitive disorders is nortriptyline. Because some of the other TCAs interact with blood pressure drugs and cause lower blood pressure, they are a risk. They may also cause a risk with patients who have heart problems. Nortriptyline, however, seems to cause fewer problems. The normal adult dosage for treating depression is 25 milligrams three or four times per day. Most elderly patients are given 30 to 50 milligrams of this drug daily, much lower than a younger adult would receive. Nortriptyline can take two to four weeks to reach its full potential in the body.

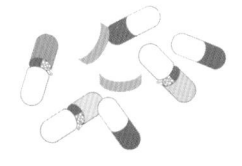

As with all drugs, treatment with TCAs should always include regular evaluation by the physician. If after a month of treatment the patient is having positive results, the medication is usually continued for a few months. At that point, the patient and physician may choose to use the TCA every other night. Finally the patient will use the drug only as needed, such as when the patient has not been sleeping well for a few nights in a row or when she is experiencing other stresses from her disease.

Effexor and Serzone are two new antidepressants which inhibit the uptake of serotonin and norepinephrine. For elderly patients, Serzone is started at 100 milligrams twice a day, half the recommended starting dose for a younger patient. As with all medications, elderly patients need to be closely monitored while taking Effexor or Serzone.

TREATMENT WITH ANTIANXIETY MEDICATIONS

Antianxiety drugs often produce immediate results; most people feel better within hours of taking their first dose. The

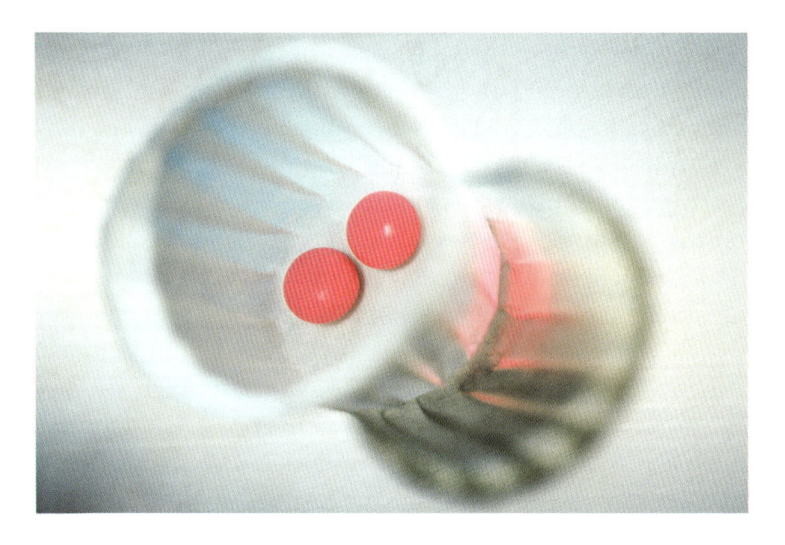

Elderly patients should take a lower dose from what a younger person would.

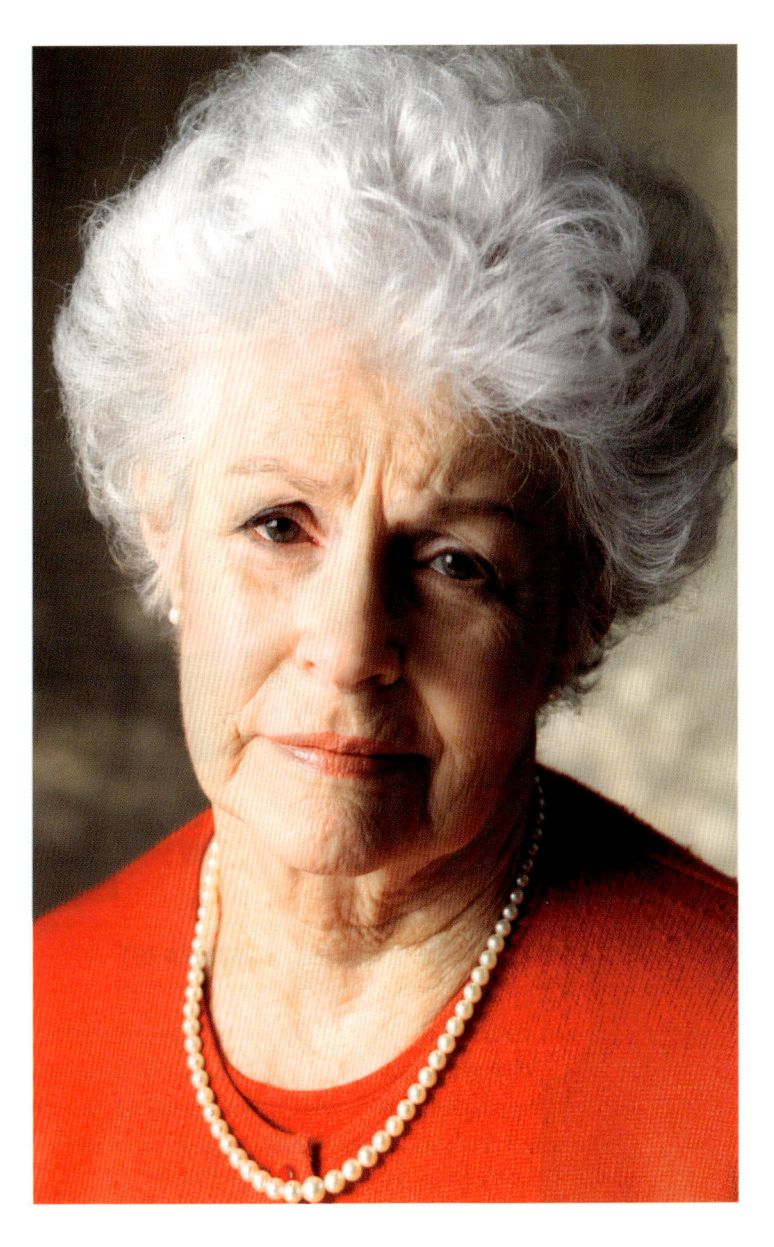

Medication can help the anxiety experienced by many people with a cognitive disorder.

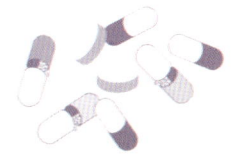

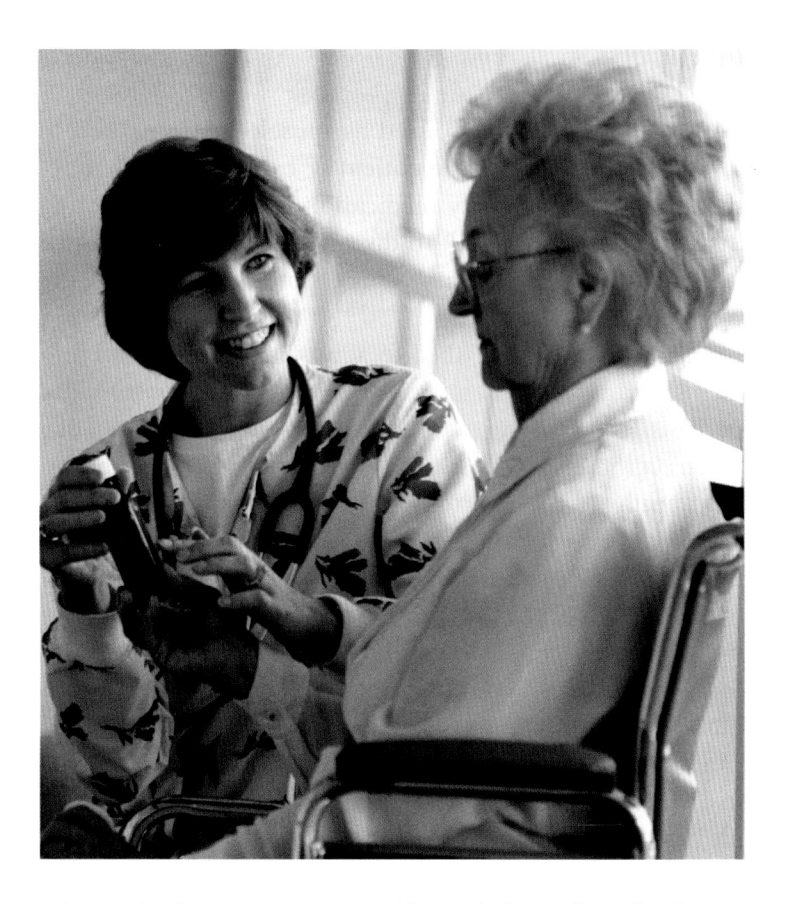

The medical practitioner should carefully explain the dosage instructions when prescribing a medication to someone with a cognitive disorder.

lower dose. Two other antipsychotic drugs that work well for older people are fluphenazine and Stelazine. Fluphenazine can be given to adult patients in split doses, 2.5 to 10 milligrams each day. The daily dose can be increased up to 20 milligrams per day. For patients with hallucinations, Stelazine should be started at 2 to 5 milligrams given twice a day; the daily dose can be increased to 15 to 20 milligrams per day. However, an elderly person may be helped with as little as one half to one quarter of the normal adult dose.

SUMMARY

A correct diagnosis is the first step toward any treatment plan. Elderly people should receive lower drug doses than younger adults; a physician should carefully monitor anyone who receives drug therapy. Drug treatment will not totally heal any cognitive disorder, but it can address many of the symptoms and allow these individuals to live happier and more satisfying lives.

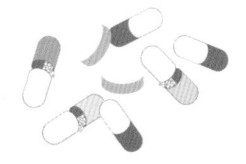

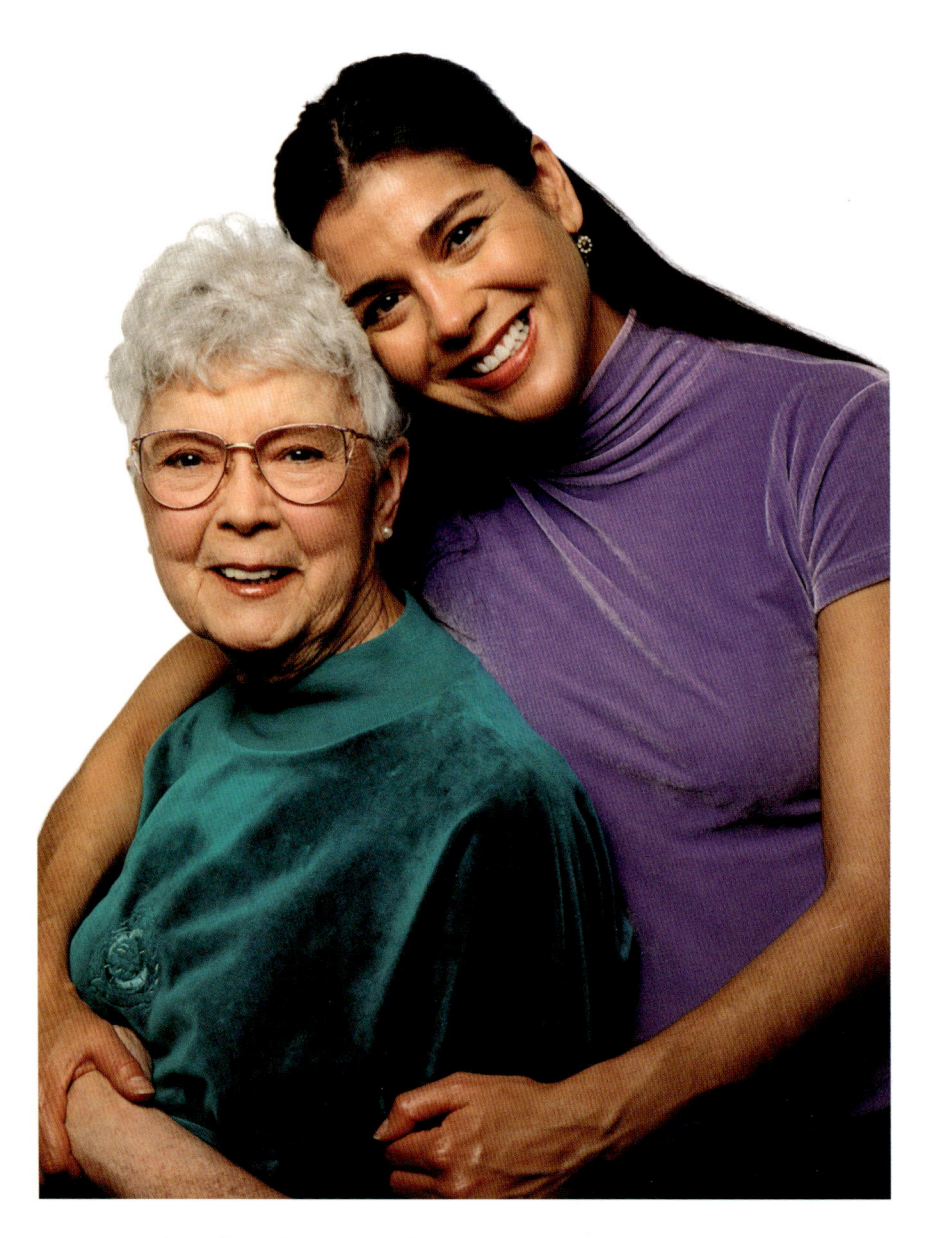

Cognitive disorders do not need to end the relationships we enjoy with loved ones.

5 | Case Histories

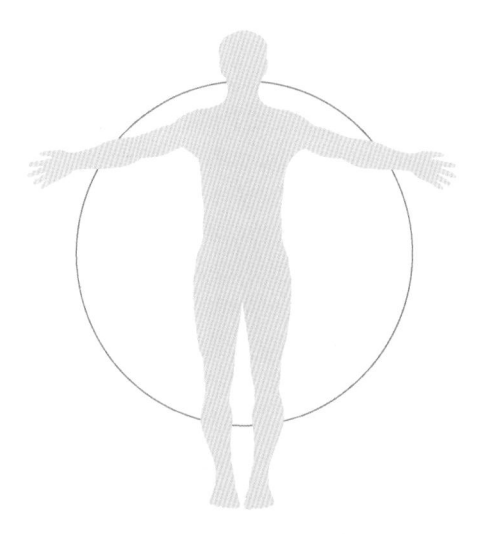

Andrea and her mother, Susanne, have always been very close. About five years ago, Andrea's dad died of a massive heart attack while at work, and since then, Susanne has grown even closer to her daughter. Andrea lives in the same neighborhood as her mother, and she enjoys visiting Susanne often.

Lately, though, Susanne seems to have more and more problems remembering things. Andrea didn't worry about it, at first. Susanna often repeated the same question twice or retold a story she had told earlier in the conversation, but this didn't seem very important to Andrea. After all, her mother was getting older, and these things were to be expected. Once in a while, Andrea had a "senior moment" of her own!

Before long, though, Andrea began noticing other changes in her mother. For one thing, Susanne was dressing differently. She had always been very conscious of her appearance and dressed each day using good taste in the makeup and jewelry she wore, even when her schedule was casual. Now, however, she wore clothes that didn't match. She often complained that she had nothing to wear, but Andrea knew she had a closet stuffed with wonderful clothes.

One day while her mother was occupied in a phone conversation with a friend, Andrea went up to her bedroom to get a book she had loaned her. She was shocked by what she found. The bedroom that had always been so neat and orderly was now a mess. Andrea moved from room to room: each room was the same. The rooms looked as if her mother had totally emptied all the closets, and the contents were strewn on the beds, dressers, and floor.

Susanne had always been an immaculate housekeeper. Andrea had noticed the downstairs was not as well kept as before, but she thought her mom was probably just letting up on her standards as she aged. Now, Andrea was seriously concerned. Something wasn't right.

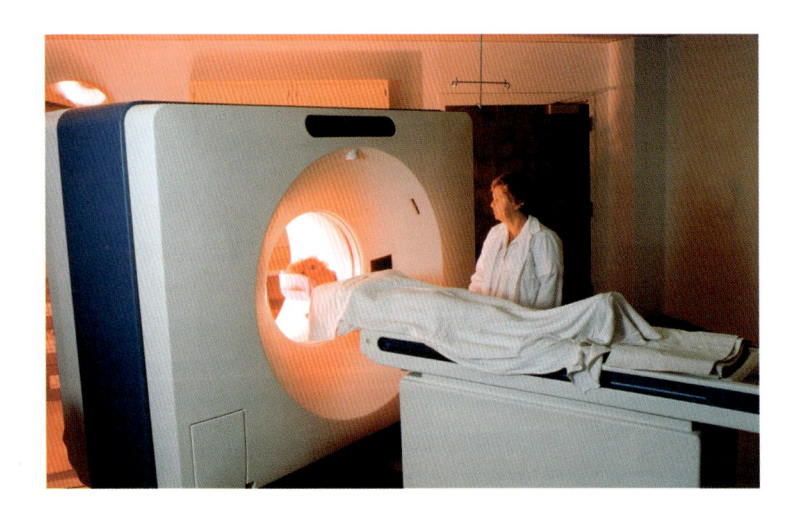

An MRI allows doctors to look at brain structures.

> Before a diagnosis can be made, tests may need to be done to make sure that some other medical condition is not creating the cognitive difficulties. These tests may include:
>
> - blood tests
> - thyroid function tests
> - tests for infectious diseases
> - tests to determine vitamin levels in the blood
> - electroencephalogram (EEG), which measures brain waves
> - electrocardiogram (ECG), which measures the electrical activity of the heart
> - cranial MRI or cranial CT scans, which look at the structures of the brain
> - spinal tap, a procedure in which a small amount of fluid is withdrawn from the spinal column to look for infection or bleeding

When Andrea asked her mother why the rooms were such a mess, Susanne just brushed her off. "I've been housecleaning, dear. Those closets are filled with stuff I just don't need any longer. I've been going through things."

Andrea accepted her mother's answer. Susanne was still handling most of her life very capably. She drove herself to her weekly quilt gathering, she took care of her banking, and she shopped for groceries. She enjoyed going to the grandchildren's after-school activities, although she insisted that Andrea call an hour before to remind her and then pick her up on the way.

One day, Andrea called to tell her mother she would be picking her up in about forty-five minutes; she reminded Susanne that they were going to a soccer game so she needed to dress warmly, since the weather was getting colder. When she arrived at her mother's house, she noticed all the windows were open. She found her mother in the kitchen baking a batch of cookies, dressed in a summer dress under a fleece coat.

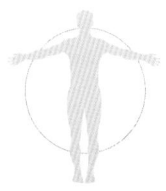

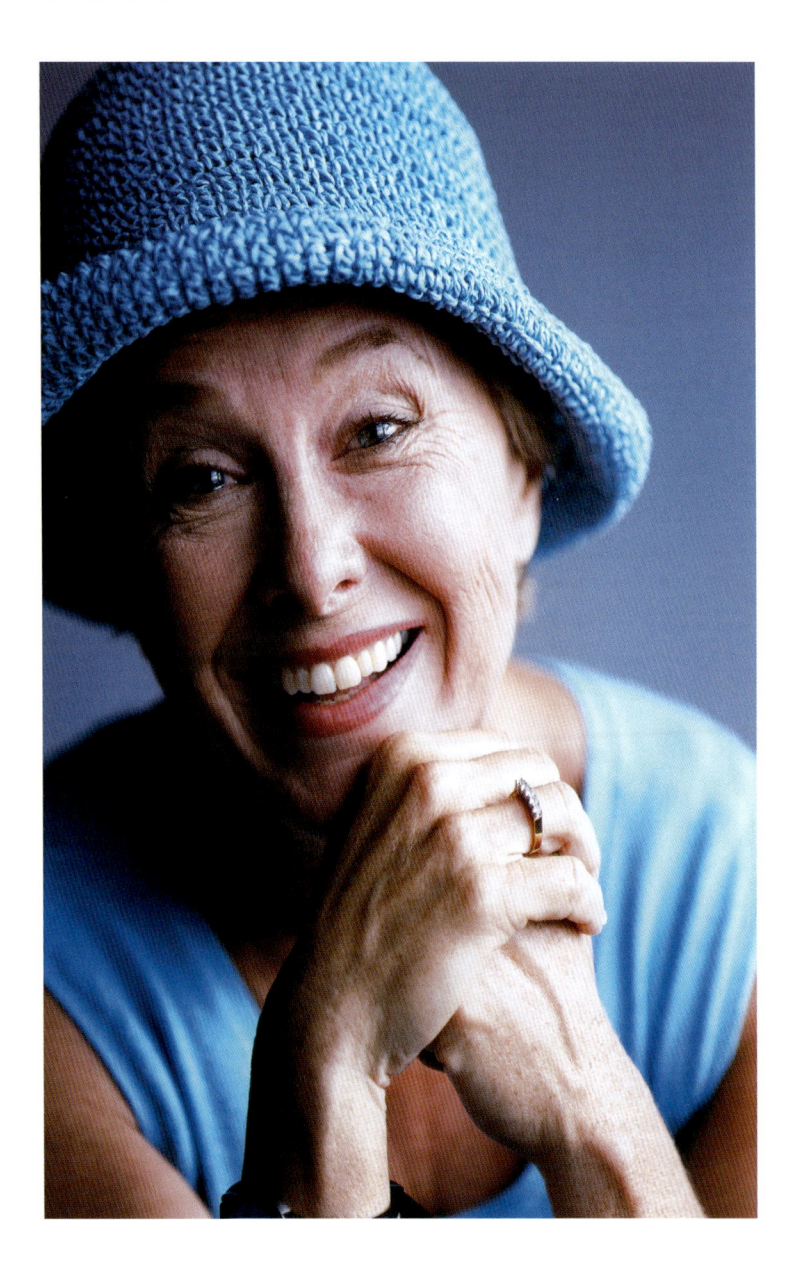

A person with a cognitive disorder will have good days as well as bad ones.

"Mother, what are you doing?" Andrea cried. "Why aren't you ready? And why do you have on a coat and why are the windows open?"

Susanne looked up from the oven. "Oh, the windows are open. I couldn't figure out why I was so cold. I *am* very cold. Where are we going, dear?"

Andrea was scared, but she still hated to accept that her mother had a definite problem. Her husband, however, talked her into taking her mother to a physician. After many tests, the doctor explained that Susanne had Alzheimer's disease.

> Alzheimer's disease research is so intense these days that many neuroscientists think the odds are good that scientists may find a way in the near future to either prevent or cure this disease completely.

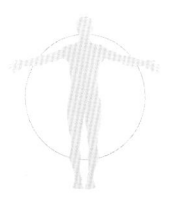

Andrea was really scared now, but her mother only shrugged. "I hate that doctor," she snapped. "I'm sure she doesn't know what she's talking about. I'm a little forgetful, but believe me, I'd know if I had Alzheimer's. I'm fine, Andrea dear. Don't you worry about me."

But Susanne's memory continued to get worse, and more and more often she did things that were out of character. Sometimes Andrea could see in Susanne's eyes that her mother understood that she was not the same. Sometimes she even said little things that indicated she knew she had Alzheimer's. But Susanne did not want to give up her home or her car. Most of the time, she stubbornly insisted she was just fine. Andrea's biggest fear now was that her mother might accidentally do something to hurt herself.

Andrea hired a health care assistant who stayed with Susanne during the day. Sometimes her mother had good days and sometimes bad; often, she treated the health care assistants so badly and complained about them so loudly that Andrea gave up and hired someone different. Eventually, though, Andrea found Doris, who loved Susanne and whom Susanne loved in return. Doris soon learned not to argue with Susanne about anything that didn't matter.

88 | CHAPTER 5

> Parkinson's disease occurs in .01 percent of the population. It is more common in elderly people, however: 1.4 percent of all people over 55 have Parkinson's and 3.4 percent of all over 75 suffer from this disease.

Sometimes he didn't even seem to recognize her, and this was most painful of all.

The doctors George and Sarah consulted treated his disease with a medication called L-dopa. Sarah could see that this drug lessened her husband's symptoms; she was relieved to resume their old loving relationship. But after being on the drug for six years, George started telling Sarah about the "little people" he saw in the hallway outside their bedroom. When they went shopping at the mall, George would sometimes stand still, staring in wonder; the people, he told Sarah, had turned into hundreds of flowers. These

> In a study conducted by neuropsychologist Yaakov Stern, the occupations of fifty-one Alzheimer's patients were rated according to memory. Stern found that those who had challenging careers involving problem solving, hard physical labor, or managing people scored much better on the memory tests than their brain scans predicted. Stern concluded that a varied yet demanding life gives a person an edge against Alzheimer's. He believes life experiences help brains overcome the damage that might cause a cognitive disorder.
>
> In a previous study, Stern had realized the value of an education in the battle against Alzheimer's, but he was surprised by the results of physical labor; exercise may also be an important factor in the prevention of this cognitive disorder. Research has also shown that vascular risk factors such as high cholesterol and high blood pressure may increase the risk for developing Alzheimer's.

Case Histories | 89

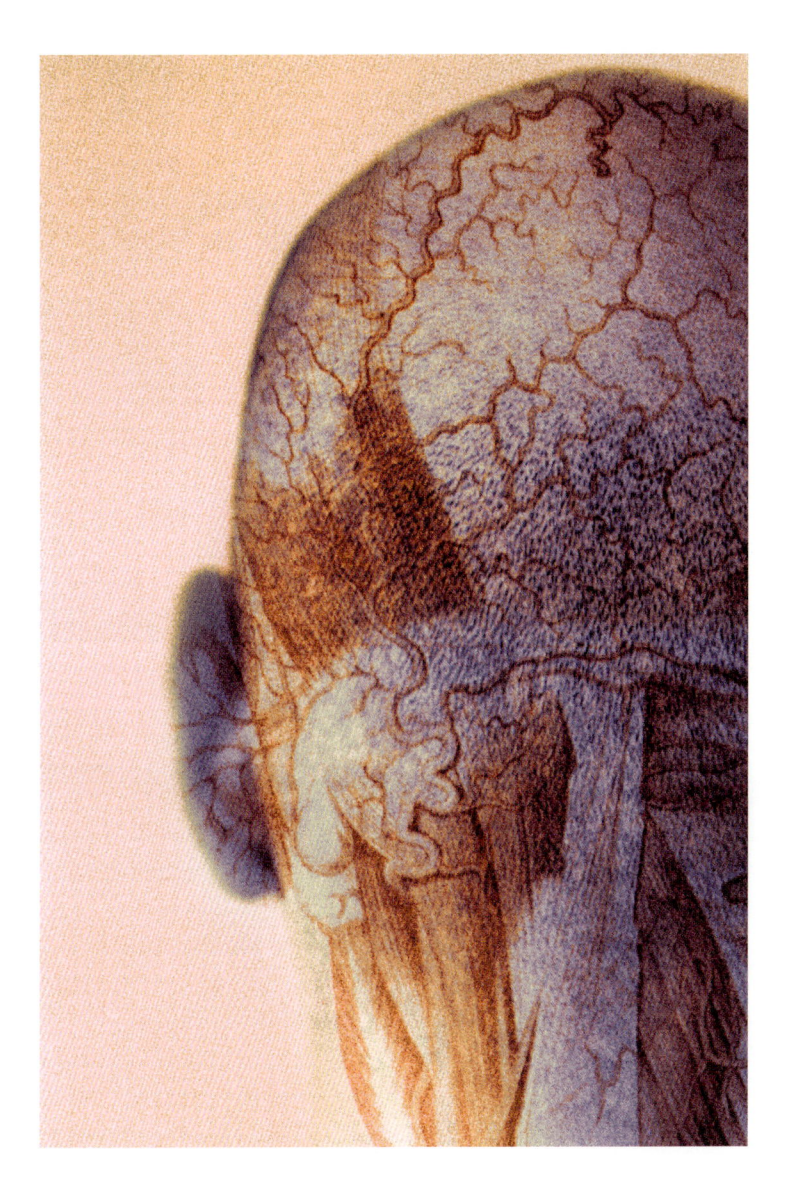

Our minds are complicated structures, connected to the rest of our bodies by nerves and blood and muscle. Mental well-being depends on total overall health—emotionally and physically.

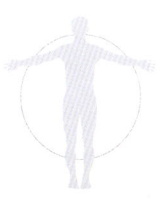

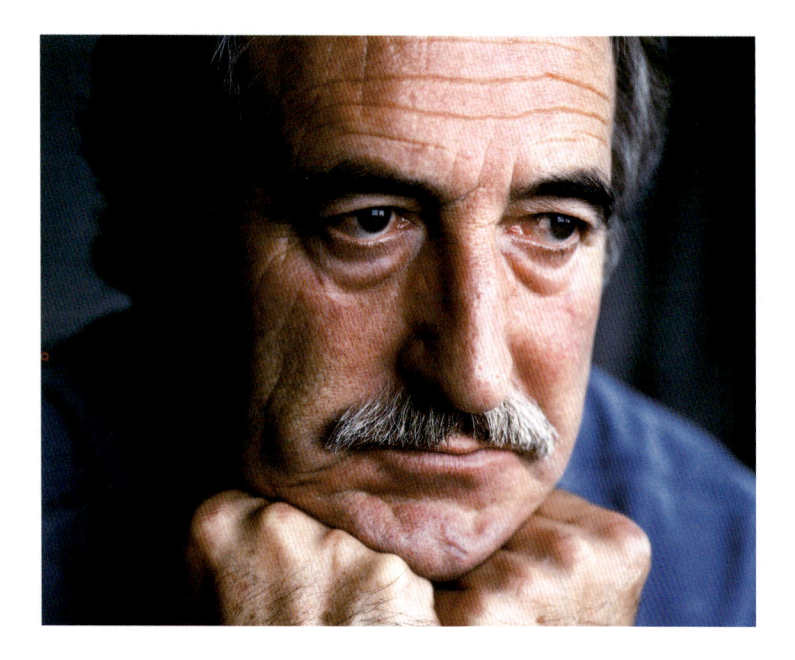

A person who is taking an antipsychotic medication may appear "zombie-like" with little emotion or expression.

hallucinations frightened Sarah, but she became even more upset when George developed delusions as well: he was convinced that Sarah was having an affair with another man. His irrational jealousy began to turn Sarah's life into a nightmare. She couldn't even go outside to get the mail without George suspecting her of meeting her lover.

The doctors decreased George's medication, and to Sarah's relief, his **psychotic** symptoms disappeared. However, his Parkinson's symptoms returned; his motor control and cognitive disorder grew noticeably worse. The doctors then changed George's drug therapy to clozapine, an antipsychotic drug. Twenty-four hours after he began taking the new drug, George was sitting in bed staring like a zombie;

> **GLOSSARY**
>
> **psychotic:** Having the characteristics of a psychosis, including a defective or lost contact with reality.

he would not speak to Sarah, he did not move, and Sarah was desperate to get back her husband.

The physicians treating George decided to try quetiapine, yet another antipsychotic medication. They started him on a dosage of 12.5 milligrams a day for the first week and then gradually increased it to 25 milligrams a day. The new treatment did not increase George's Parkinson's symptoms, and it reduced his delusions and hallucinations. Sometimes he still told Sarah about the fairy-like creatures he saw on their walks, but he understood now that these images were the effect of his disease. He no longer suspected Sarah of being unfaithful to him. Sarah was relieved to resume her loving relationship with her husband—and she was grateful he could continue to live at home with her, enjoying the same leisurely breakfasts, slow walks along the

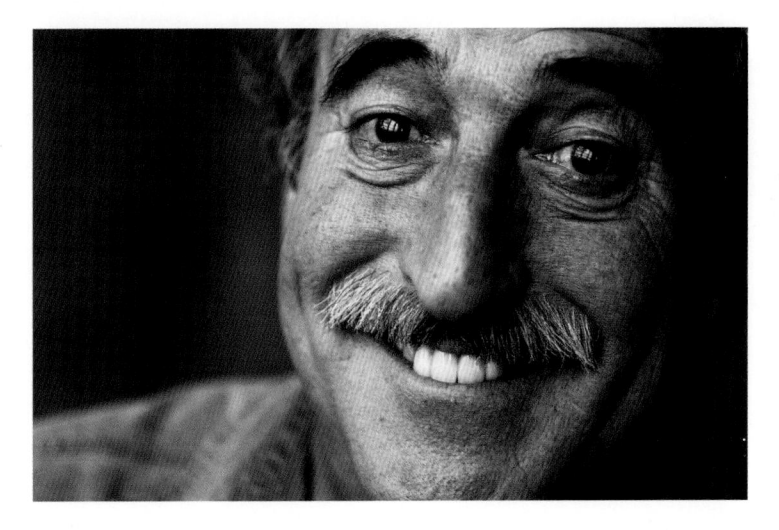

Finding the right medication at the right dosage level allows the individual to become more like his old self.

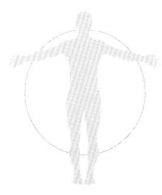

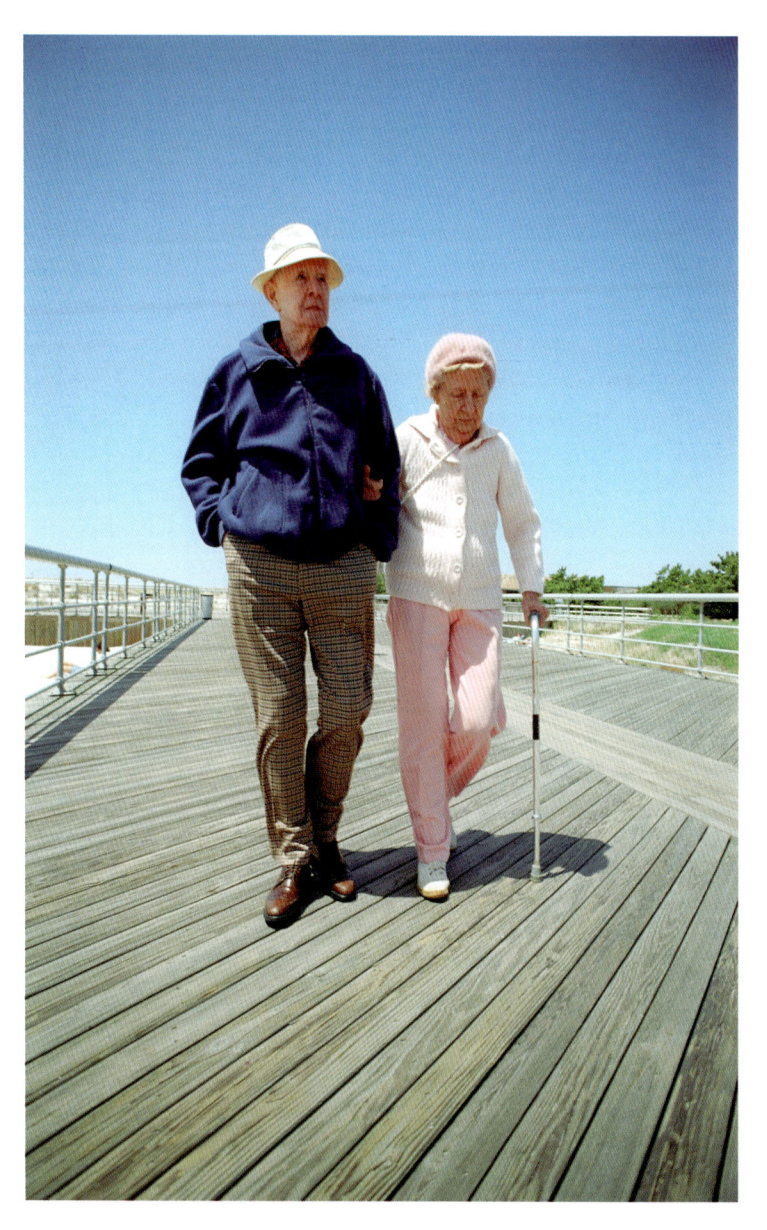

As people age, they may experience impaired mobility—but they are entitled to enjoy the same activities and relationships they have always enjoyed.

road outside their house, and relaxed afternoon gardening they had enjoyed together for years.

For people like Susanne and George, drugs offer no magic cures. They may help control the symptoms, but their side effects may sometimes be harder to bear than the original condition.

More and more researchers believe that the only hope for fighting Alzheimer's and other cognitive disorders is through prevention. Drugs offer the most hope to those like Carolyn who are in the early stages of a cognitive disorder; for these people, cognitive enhancers such as Reminyl, Aricept, and Exelon may be able to keep the disease from getting worse. For those like Susanne and George there is little hope of cure, but with the help of medications these people can lead lives that are contented and fulfilling in their own way.

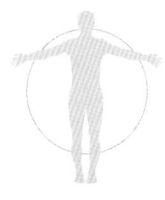

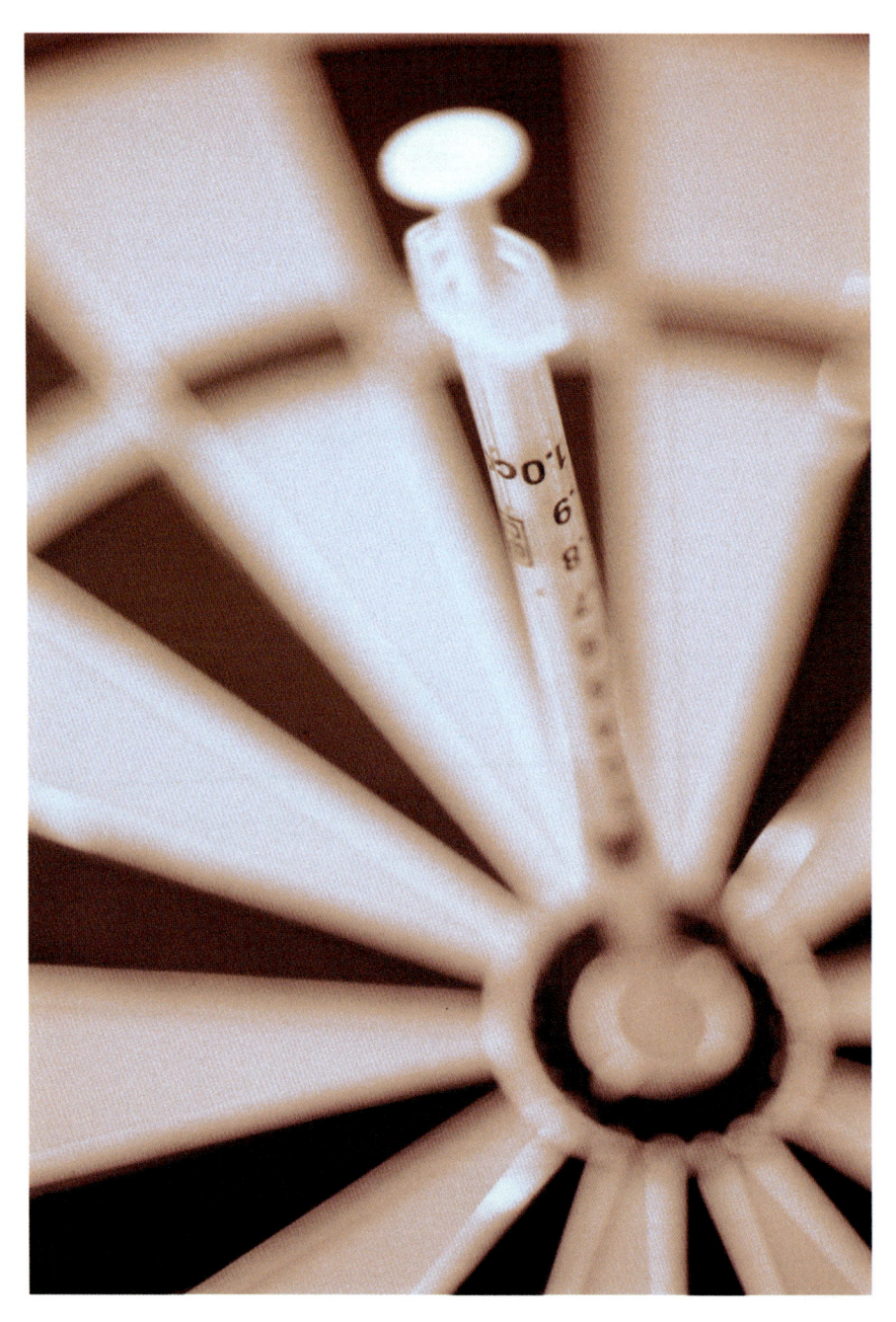

Sometimes it's hard to hit the "bull's eye" when it comes to treating a psychiatric disorder. Psychiatric drugs are powerful chemicals that can affect other parts of the body as well.

6 | Risks and Side Effects

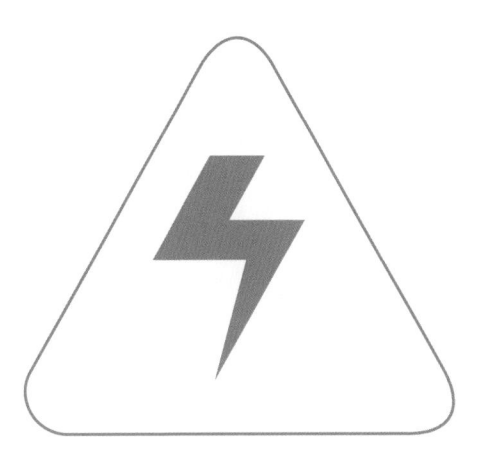

My dear grandchildren,

Once I became a part of the study, the first medication they gave me was Aricept. You may have already heard of it because it has been the most common drug used to treat Alzheimer's patients and therefore has been studied the most with patients. I tried it and began to have horrible nightmares. I rarely remembered my dreams before this, but now I began to wake every night, haunted by horrible dream images. I was soon exhausted.

I finally called the clinic and said I didn't think I could handle it. They decided to try me on another drug called Exelon. This drug gave me terrible leg cramps every night and sometimes during the day as well. I still was not sleeping and I was very tired. Being tired does not help a healthy person's memory, and things were even worse for me.

I am now on a third medication called Reminyl. I started on a low dose. As I have tolerated it, the dose has been in-

creased. At first the drug made me nauseated, but I kept taking it anyway. Gradually, it bothered me less and less, and as I have gotten used to the drug, the dosage has been increased little by little.

I go to the clinic for a checkup about every three months now, and once a year there is a full-day session like my first one. It would be wonderful to say "I am being cured!" But with this disease, the only hope so far is that medicine can keep a patient from deteriorating further.

I'm holding on to that hope. I want to enjoy you children for as long as I can.

*Love,
Nana Carolyn*

Hope is what keeps patients such as Carolyn open to trying different drugs and to being involved with studies like the one in which she is participating. It is also hope that keeps scientists looking for answers to the many unanswered questions of MCI and Alzheimer's disease. As researchers look for answers, they need the participation of patients in testing drugs. Testing helps scientists understand how the disease affects patients and how the drugs work to affect the disease. Understanding the side effects caused by these drugs is an essential part of the research process.

One of the problems of treating persons with a cognitive disorder is that some of the drugs that might help relieve symptoms may also cause further memory loss and cognitive impairment. Some of these include antihistamines, tranquilizers, sedatives, narcotics, antacids, some antidepressants, and even certain blood pressure medications such as beta-blockers and calcium channel blockers.

Another important consideration doctors must keep in mind when working with the elderly is their sensitivity to

Risks and Side Effects | 97

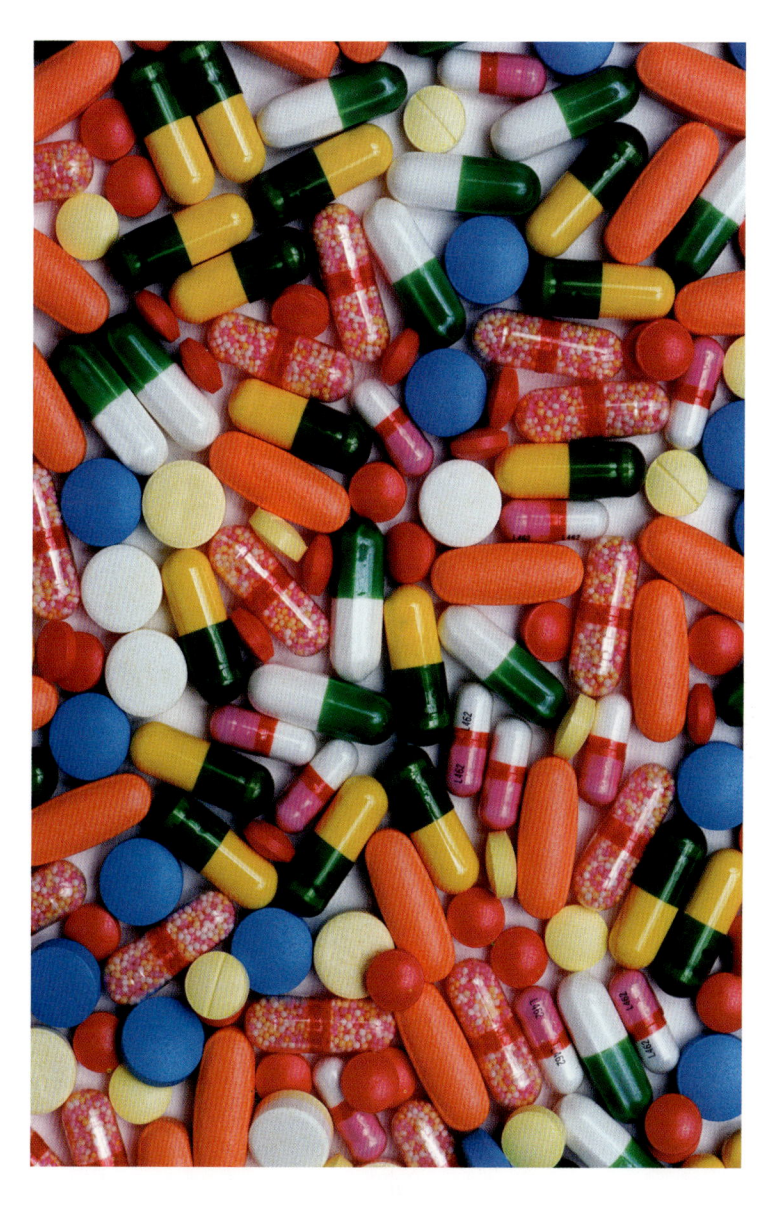

Medications offer hope to people with cognitive disorders—but understanding drugs' side effects is an essential element of treatment.

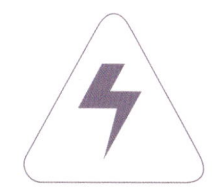

GLOSSARY

anorexia: *An eating disorder characterized by the inability or refusal to maintain a minimum weight.*

impotence: *The inability to achieve or maintain an erect penis.*

SIDE EFFECTS OF COGNITIVE ENHANCERS

Carolyn's experience with the cognitive enhancers like Reminyl, Aricept, and Exelon is not unusual. These drugs often cause nausea, vomiting, or diarrhea. They may sometimes also cause weight loss and ***anorexia.*** Experimentation with these various drugs and their dosage levels may allow doctors to determine a treatment whose benefits outweigh the risks. In some cases, however, particularly in more advanced cases of cognitive disorders, the discomfort caused by the drugs will not be perceived by the patient and her family as being worth the possible benefits.

Tacrine, as we mentioned in an earlier chapter, is no longer prescribed as often as the newer cognitive enhancers. The risk of liver damage is often perceived to be too great.

SIDE EFFECTS OF ANTIDEPRESSANTS

SSRIs

Not everyone taking the SSRI antidepressants experiences side effects, but for some people, mild side effects such as difficulty sleeping, anxiety, weakness, tremors, sweating, ***impotence***, nausea, drowsiness, dizziness, stomach upset, weight gain, nervousness, or yawning may be a problem when they first take an antidepressant like Prozac or Zoloft. In many cases, these annoyances will go away within a few weeks and may not be serious enough to give reason to stop taking the medication. For others, the side effects can be severe enough that the discomfort of the side effect outweighs the effectiveness of the drug.

About one in twelve patients taking Prozac develop an itching rash. This can be a serious side effect that causes about one third of the persons taking this drug to discon-

Risks and Side Effects | 101

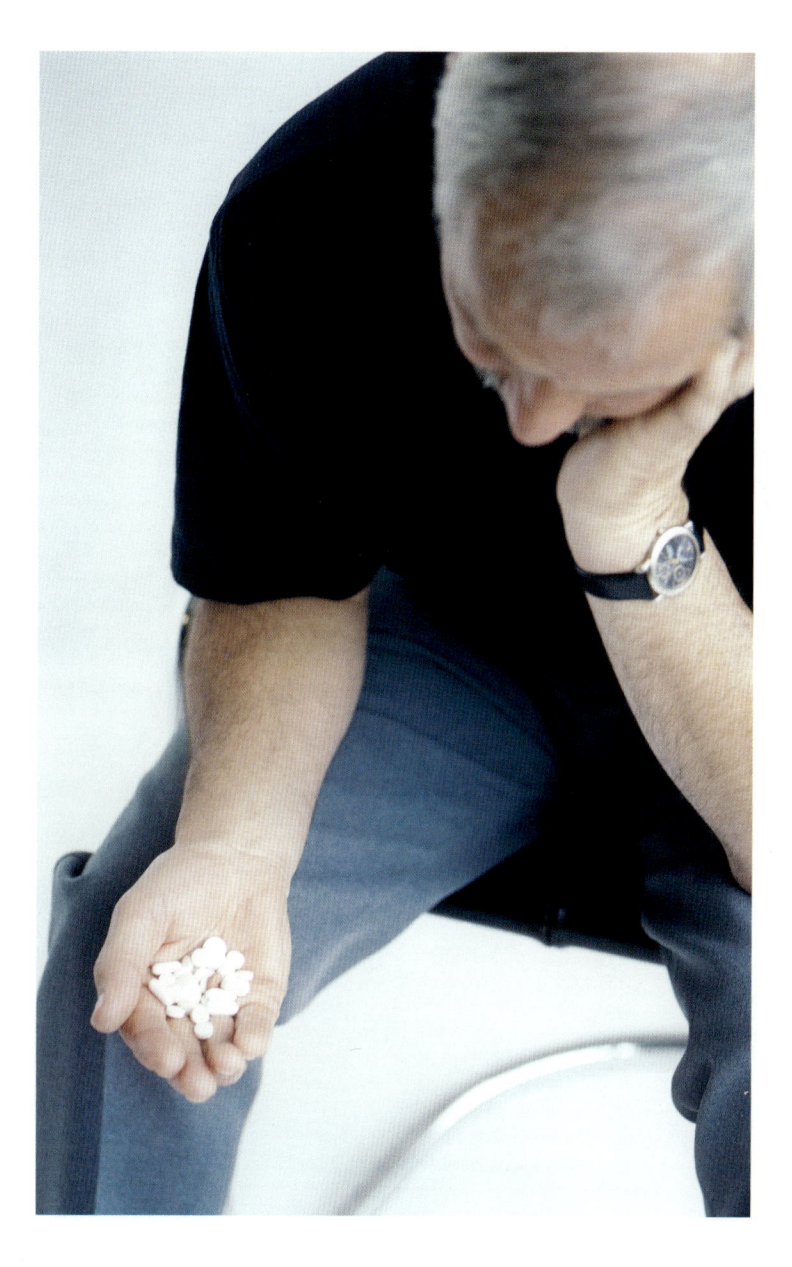

Some people who take an SSRI may experience weakness or drowsiness.

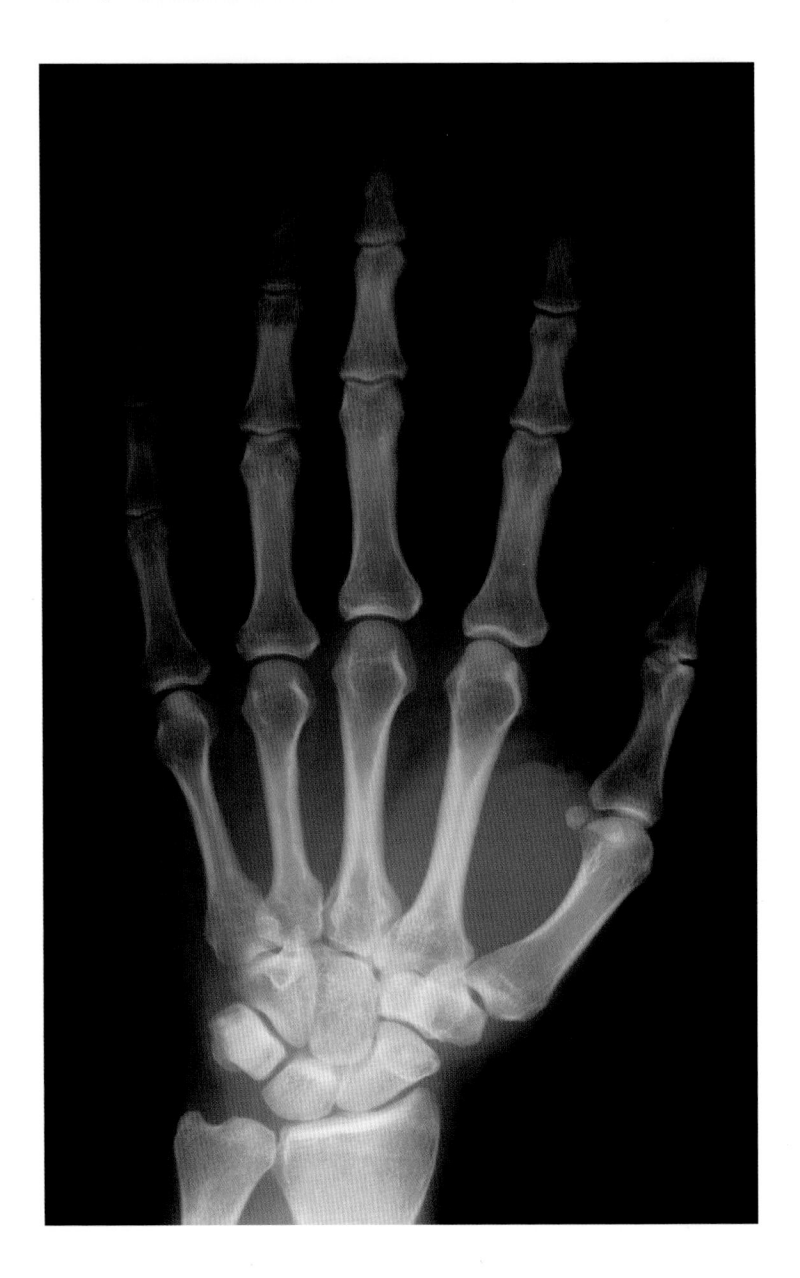

Prozac can cause joint pain.

> **Precautions for Taking Zoloft and Prozac**
>
> 1. Always inform your doctor of any other prescription or over-the-counter medications that you are taking.
> 2. Consuming alcoholic beverages is not recommended.
> 3. Caution should be taken when using:
>   Diazepam for antianxiety and sedative treatment
>   Digoxin for heart treatment
>   lithium for manic-depressive and bipolar treatment
>   other psychiatric antidepressants such as Elavil
>   over-the-counter cold remedies
>   Warfarin, an anticoagulant
> 4. Serious and possibly fatal reactions can occur when taking a monoamine oxidase inhibitor (MAOI) such as Nardil, Parnate, and Marplan. Allow 14 days between discontinuing MAOI therapy and beginning Zoloft or Prozac.
> 5. A rash can be the sign of a serious medical condition for those taking Prozac. See your physician immediately if you develop a rash while taking the medication.
> 6. Alert your physician to any reactions to other antidepressants.

tinue the medication. Other symptoms that may appear with the rash are fever, joint pain, swelling, wrist and hand pain, breathing difficulties, swollen lymph glands, and some laboratory test abnormalities. Most people have no further problems once they stop taking the drug and begin appropriate antihistamine or corticosteroid therapy.

Because SSRIs are broken down in the liver, patients with liver disease must use caution when taking the drug, using lower doses at the start of the drug therapy or trying some other drug. SSRIs also affect blood platelets, blood cells important in the coagulation or thickening of the blood. Because of this effect, some patients have experienced abnormal bleeding while using the drug. This relatively rare symptom should be shared with the physician immediately.

Some SSRIs can cause serious side effects when combined with other medications. The doctor or pharmacist should be consulted before taking any additional drugs, including over-the-counter or natural medications.

Caution should be used until the correct dose has been determined. Although SSRIs do not normally act like a sedative, some people may notice some sedative qualities when first taking the drug. This usually goes away after a short time. People who are elderly or suffering from the motor symptoms of Parkinson's disease should be watched carefully to ensure they do not fall. As has been mentioned before, medication affects each person differently.

Tricyclic Antidepressants

Drowsiness is the most common side effect of the TCAs, but about 10 to 15 percent of the patients taking these drugs will become "hyper" or agitated instead. Other common side effects include dry mouth, blurred vision, constipation, low blood pressure, and heart palpitations.

As with any medication that alters body functions, antidepressants must be monitored by a physician. Finding the right doctor and keeping him aware of any changes experienced while taking an SSRI or TCA is the best way to eliminate the concern over side effects. Both a slow start-up and a slow discontinuation help protect patients from unnecessary problems.

SIDE EFFECTS OF ANTIANXIETY DRUGS

Although benzodiazepines can be beneficial when treating anxiety in those who have cognitive disorders, these drugs' addictive quality can be problematic. Weaning from low doses after taking the drug for only a few weeks usually only causes sleep problems or anxiety, symptoms that may have caused the patient to take the drug initially. But for those who have developed a dependence on this chemical (which may happen after only four weeks of regular use), discontinuing the drug may cause symptoms that include sensitivity to bright lights, sleep disturbances, tremors, twitching, poor concentration, flu-like symptoms, and appetite loss. Those who have taken the drug for long periods of time and decide to terminate their use may experience tremors, weakness, and even seizures, delirium, depression, or death. As a re-

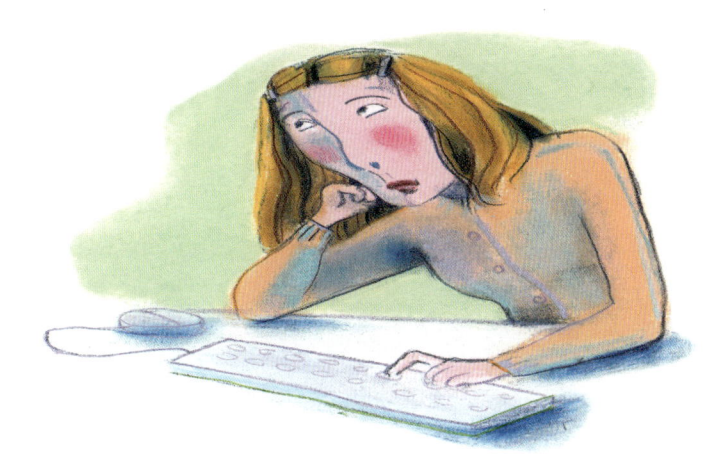

A person taking a benzodiazepine may have difficulty concentrating.

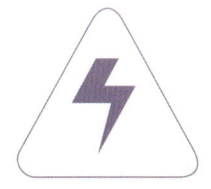

106 | CHAPTER 6

sult, the patient, family, and physician must carefully weigh whether the risks of anxiety outweigh the medication's risks.

While using these drugs, the side effects are usually minimal. There may be mild drowsiness for the first few days, and sometimes the elderly become weak and confused. However, side effects generally become more prevalent when high doses are used over long periods of time. These side effects include headaches, irritability, confusion, memory loss, and depression.

Some medical conditions can increase the risk factors

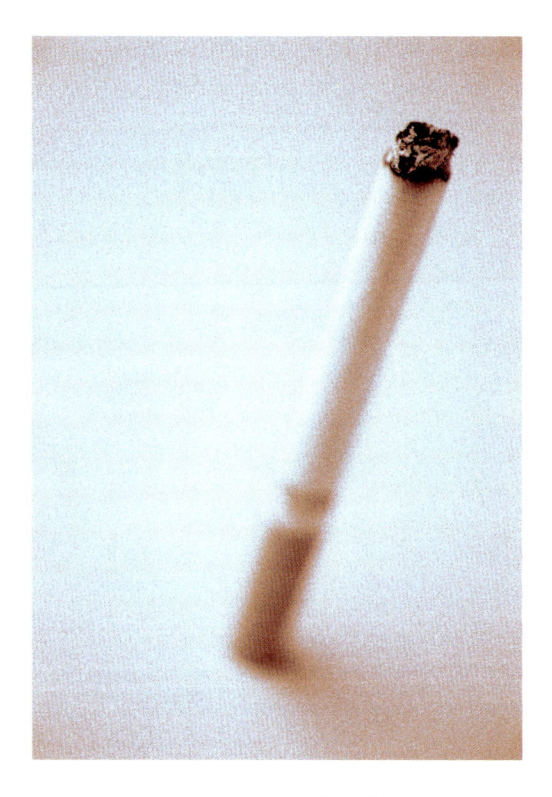

Smoking cigarettes may decrease the effectiveness of antianxiety medications.

for using an antianxiety medication. Caution should be used when taking a benzodiazepine if the person suffers from severe depression, severe lung disease, sleep apnea, alcohol problems, and kidney disease. Alcohol should be avoided, along with other tranquilizers, narcotics, barbiturates, antihistamines, and antidepressants; death can occur when antianxiety medications are used along with alcohol and other drugs. Smoking can decrease the effectiveness of the drug.

SUMMARY

Some people with cognitive disorders are afraid to take medication. They fear that the drugs will damage their brains even more; they worry that they will feel "drugged" and even more confused than they are already. Drugs are powerful chemicals that can have complicated effects on the brain, so these are realistic concerns. However, when a physician carefully monitors the use of these drugs, they can give real help to people with cognitive disorders. People like Carolyn should not live in fear and hopelessness if they don't have to.

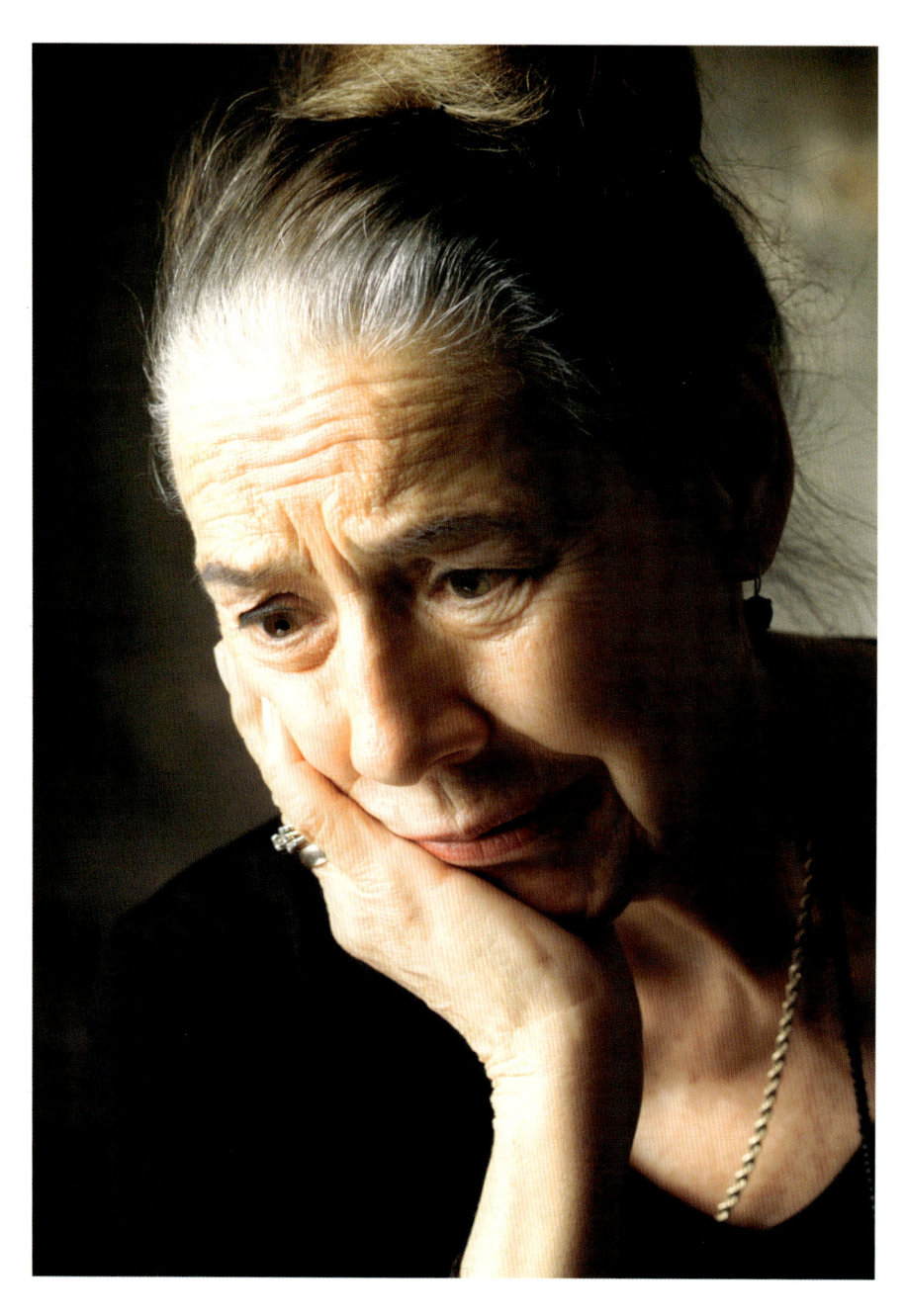

A person with a cognitive disorder may wrestle with loneliness and depression.

7 | Alternative Treatment

My dear grandchildren,

I know I'm not the only one to run into mood swings and other worries as I try to deal with the changes in my life. You kids have your own troubles, too. Do you ever feel as though no one, not even your family and your friends, really understands you? You may wonder if anyone really cares, and you may wish you could explain how you are feeling to someone else. I feel that way often.

Grandpa has been very kind and wonderful to me, but sometimes I just wish I could talk to another person who is going through the same stuff I am. As a therapist, I have often led support groups for people with drug and alcohol problems. These groups often included members' families and friends, and I have always found that people can best share and relate to each other when they know other people feel just like they do. It really helps when you can talk with other people who are experiencing a lot of the same frustrations or fears you are.

One of the hardest things for me is that there are no support groups, at least in my area, for people who have a cognitive disorder. There are now many groups for people who are caregivers of Alzheimer's patients—and these people definitely need support and understanding to help them cope with their lives. Sometimes, though, I feel like asking, "But what about me? Why isn't there a group to help me?*" I feel so lonely and "different," as though I'm the only person in the world who is going through this. Sometimes I could explode because I feel so angry . . . and sometimes I just wish someone would cry with me and hold me. It is easy to become depressed when you think no one really understands.*

But I'm glad for you children, because I know you will try to understand what I'm going through. Your love means a lot to me. Even though you are only children, never forget how much power you have. When you take the time to show me your love, you make my life easier.

With love,
Nana Carolyn

PSYCHOTHERAPY

Medication alone will never be enough to help those suffering from a cognitive disorder. Carolyn's feelings of fear, anger, and depression are very normal when faced with circumstances like this. When drug therapy is supplemented with some form of ***psychotherapy,*** individuals like Carolyn no longer feel so alone.

Support groups are one form of psychotherapy that offer a place where emotions, fears, and real questions can be openly expressed. In order to work well, these groups should be directed by a mental health professional who pro-

> **GLOSSARY**
>
> **psychotherapy:** A treatment of mental or emotional disorders. Sometimes called talking therapy.

Alternative Treatment | 111

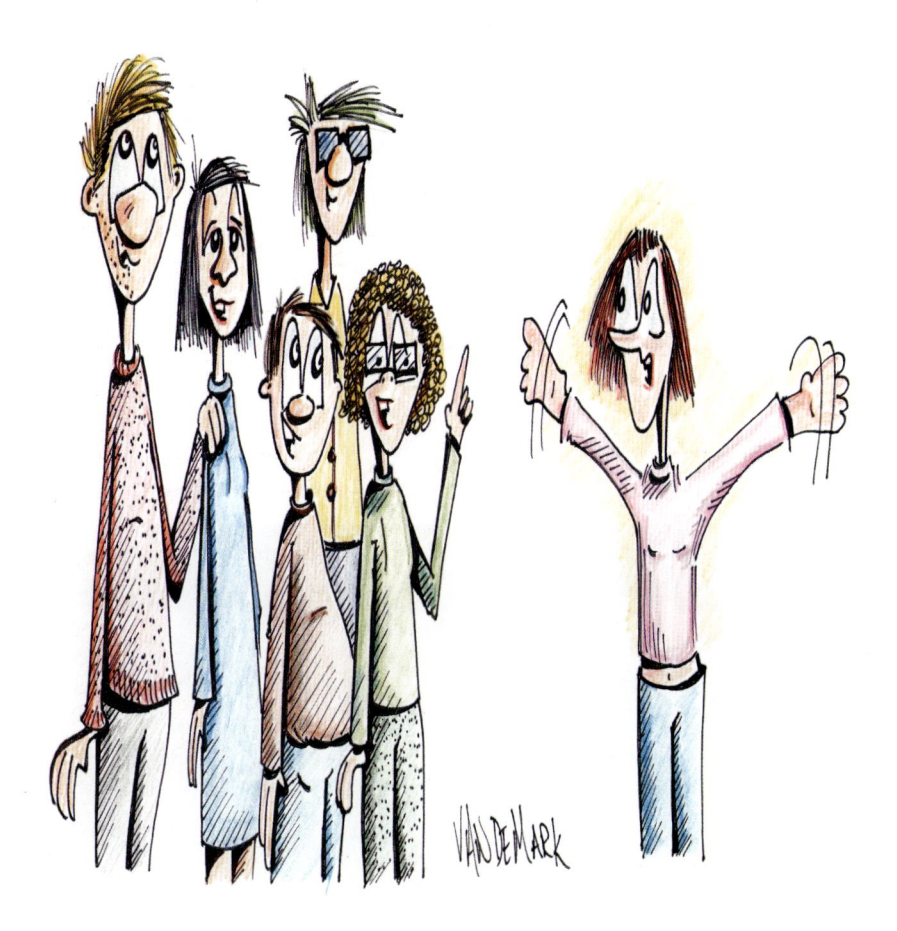

A person with a cognitive disorder may feel that no one else truly understands what she is trying to communicate.

112 | CHAPTER 7

vides guided support. Because of the leader's knowledge, the group experiences peer support and can learn new coping strategies, problem-solving skills, and information about new studies and medications.

VITAMIN THERAPY

Studies have been done on the importance of vitamin E as a supplement for Alzheimer's patients. In the Alzheimer's Disease Cooperative Study, for example, a dose of 1,000 IU of vitamin E and 5 milligrams of selignine twice daily delayed nursing home placement, loss of the ability to perform self-care, and severe dementia. Vitamin E may help the brain cells defend themselves against damage by free radicals. Formed as a by-product of normal cell function, free radi-

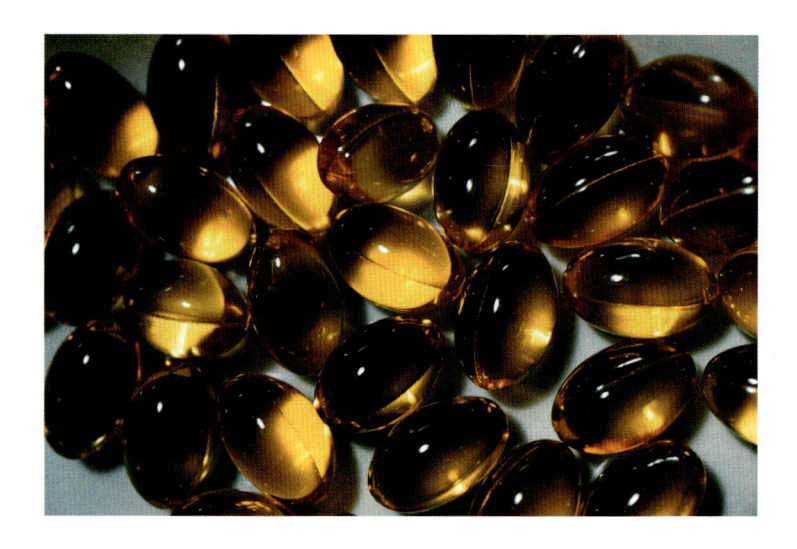

Vitamin E may help protect the brain from further damage.

> ### Homeopathic Treatment for Cognitive Disorders
>
> Homeopathy is a form of alternative medicine that treats disease and disorders from a very different perspective from conventional medicine. It looks at a person's entire physical and mental being, rather than dividing a patient into various symptoms and disorders. Homeopathic medicine uses tiny doses to stimulate the body's ability to heal itself. In some cases, these doses may be administered only once every few months or years.
>
> According to Judyth Reichenberg-Ullman and Robert Ullman, authors of *Prozac Free: Homeopathic Medicine for Depression, Anxiety, and Other Mental and Emotional Problems*, homeopathy offers safe, natural alternatives that can supplement or replace conventional pharmaceutical treatment. They recommend this form of treatment because it has fewer side effects than conventional drugs. Homeopathic treatment should always be administered by a licensed homeopathic practitioner.

cals are a kind of oxygen molecule that can damage cell structure. Some believe they have a role in Alzheimer's disease. For this reason, many physicians and researchers look at the effects of vitamin E to build up cell defense naturally. Some precautions should be used in taking vitamin E, though. It may interfere with blood thinning medications and too much of it may be toxic. As with other medications, taking vitamin E should be monitored by a physician.

Herbs are powerful medicines and should be treated as such.

- Never use herbs to self-treat for serious medical conditions or persistent symptoms.
- Don't use herbs in place of medicines prescribed by a healthcare provider.
- Never take more than the recommended dosage of any herbal preparation.
- Start with low dosages because it's not uncommon to be sensitive to herbs.
- Tell your health-care provider and pharmacist about any herbal remedies being taken.
- Stop taking an herb right away if there are any side effects.
- Report side effects immediately to the health-care provider and to the FDA's Med Watch line at 1-800-332-1088.
- Choose products that give the Latin botanical name and the quantity of herb contained in them.

HERBAL THERAPY

Ginkgo Biloba

Researchers in Europe believe that a large body of evidence suggests that the herb ginkgo biloba will help to boost memory and brain function. German researchers have found that giving ginkgo biloba to people who have been diagnosed with memory problems significantly improves their memory skills after only six weeks. In other tests carried out on elderly patients who all had difficulty remembering things, doses of 120 milligrams of ginkgo biloba a day were found to benefit cognitive (learning and memory) function within three months. American researchers do not always agree with these results, however, and the U.S. Food

Alternative Treatment | 115

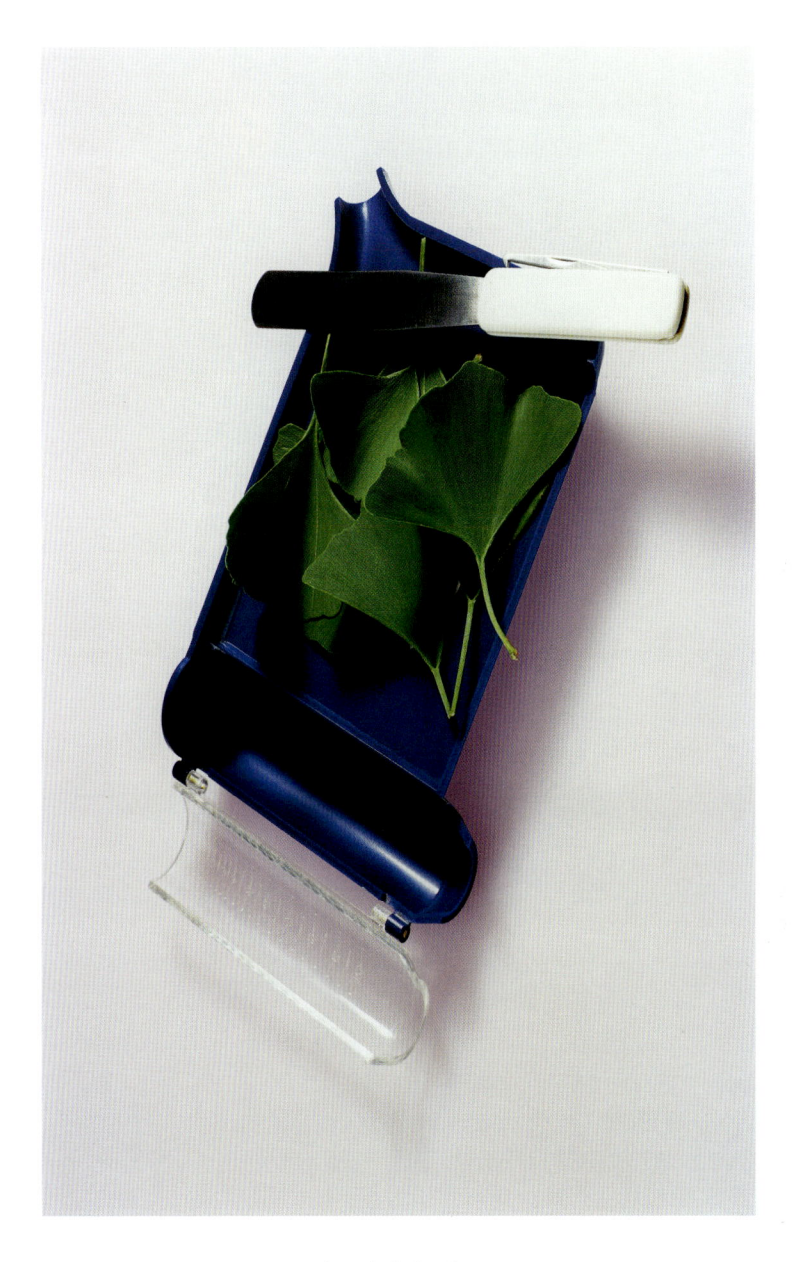

Ginkgo biloba leaves.

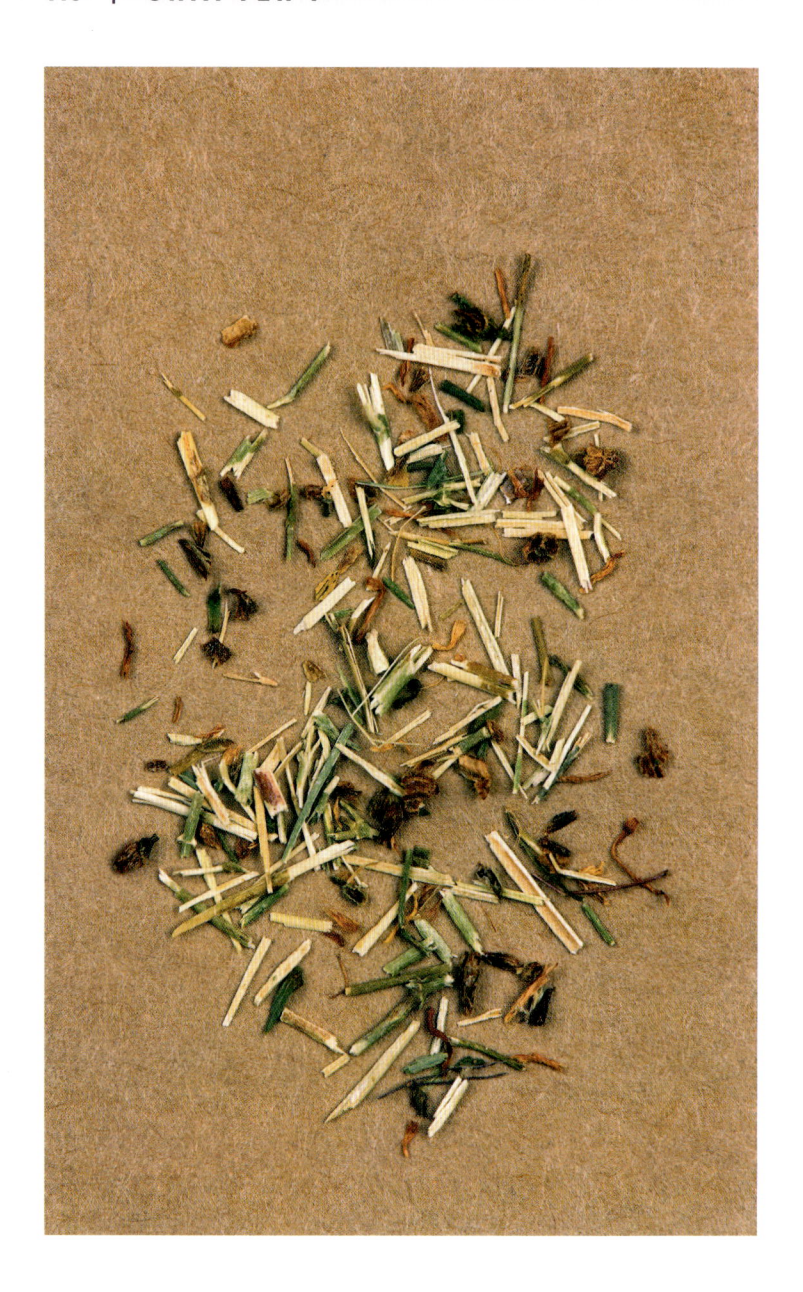

Saint-John's-wort is an herbal remedy used to treat depression.

> The American Society of Anesthesiologists cautions that herbs can interact with medicines used before, during, and after surgery. A recent study focusing on the effects of echinacea, ephedra, garlic, ginkgo, ginseng, kava, Saint-John's-wort, and valerian determined that it is best to stop taking all herbal remedies at least two weeks before planned surgery. Any herbal remedies taken should be mentioned to the surgeon and anesthesiologist.

and Drug Administration has not approved ginkgo biloba as a cognitive enhancer.

Butcher's Broom

Butcher's broom contains anti-inflammatory properties and has the ability to improve the structure of the veins. This herb may improve brain function by increasing the blood supply to brain cells.

Kelp

Kelp is a sea vegetable high in mineral content, especially iodine and potassium. This vegetable is thought to increase thyroid function and prevent absorption of radiation and heavy metals. (Some people believe that these heavy metals are one cause of Alzheimer's disease.) Kelp is said to be beneficial for sensory nerves, the brain, spinal tissues, and membranes.

OTHER TREATMENTS

Mild memory loss comes normally with aging, but keeping the brain active may help to preserve brain cells. Reading,

118 | **CHAPTER 7**

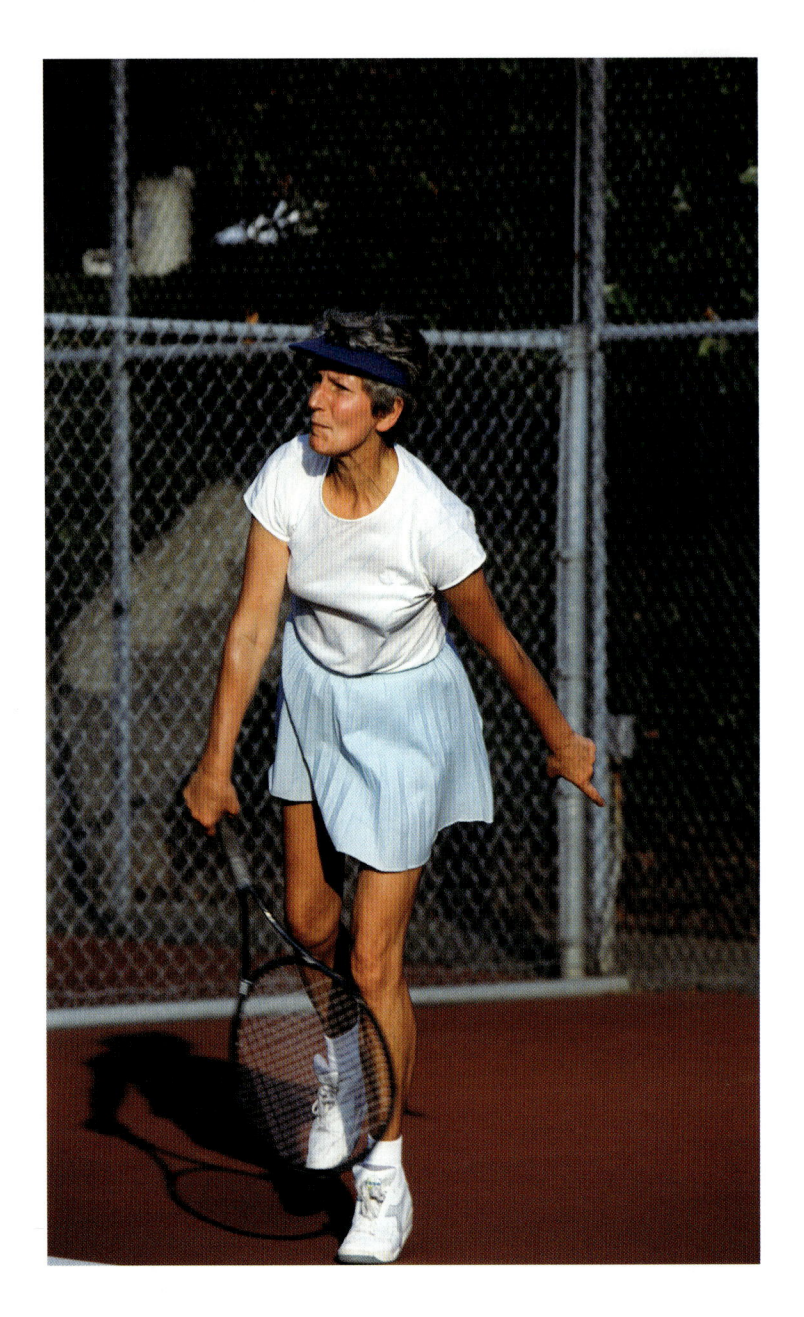

Exercise stimulates the flow of blood to the brain.

Alternative Treatment | 119

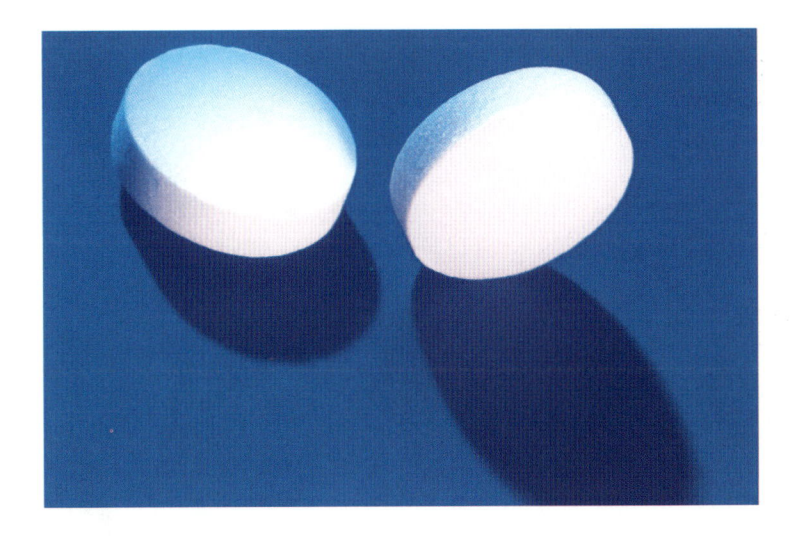

Low doses of aspirin may reduce memory loss.

singing, doing puzzles, conversing, exercising, and eating a balanced diet stimulate blood flow and may increase cell connections in the brain.

Researchers have found other medications that may slow the progress of Alzheimer's disease and other cognitive disorders. For instance, low doses of aspirin and nonsteroidal anti-inflammatory drugs (NSAIDs) may reduce memory loss by making blood cells and vessels less sticky and improving blood flow. Hormone replacement therapy for menopausal women may delay the onset of symptoms of Alzheimer's disease. The relationship between the hormone estrogen and Alzheimer's disease still needs further investigation.

FAMILY SUPPORT

Clearly, the support Carolyn receives from her husband is very important to her; she has come to rely on him a great

How to Stay Sharp

You can protect and improve your memory. Here are a few tips:

- Learn new skills, especially something different from your normal activities. (For instance, learn to dance if you work at a computer all day.)
- Concentrate on important facts. (For example, hold a pen in your hand and think about its characteristics, including what it is made of, its function, its color, and its various parts. Don't think about anything else while you are concentrating on the pen.)
- Relax. (You cannot pay attention to important things while you are tense or nervous.)
- Use coding skills to associate facts to images so that they can be more readily recalled later. (For example, if you needed to remember that a man's name was Mr. Drummond, you could visualize him playing a drum.)
- Think of visual images. (Imagine a big slice of pizza. Smell the melted cheese and sauce and feel the crust in your hand. Imagine taking a bite and seeing the cheese string between your mouth and the slice. If your mouth filled with saliva while you visualized this scene, then your visualization is successful. Now try an ice cream sundae or chocolate cake.)
- Eat plenty of foods with thiamine, folic acid, and B_{12}. (These memory-improving vitamins are found in bread, cereal, vegetables, and fruits.)
- Drink plenty of water to help maintain memory systems. (Some physicians believe that a lack of water has an immediate and deep effect on memory. When someone becomes dehydrated, he usually suffers from confusion and other thought problems.)
- Get enough sleep. (The brain disconnects from the senses during sleep and is able to revise and store memory.)
- Be aware that some medications such as tranquilizers, muscle relaxants, and sleeping pills, as well as alcohol and smoking, can cause memory problems.
- Keep physically fit.
- Take notes, get organized, and use a diary to help your memory.

Adapted from Silvia Helena Cardoso, *Brain and Mind*.

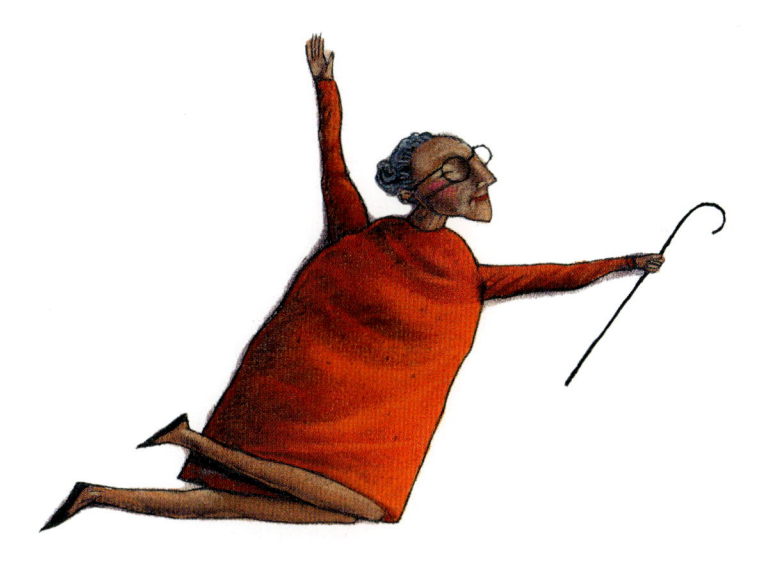

We are each different, and we each age differently—but life has much joy for us all to experience, no matter how old we are.

deal. Her dependency is bound to change the nature of their relationship, but Carolyn and her husband may find that although these changes are difficult, they also bring their own rewards.

Family members need to learn and accept how their loved one changes throughout the disease. Each person's experience will be different; no "book knowledge" can replace simply being "tuned in" to the individual, listening to her concerns, paying attention to her symptoms, and validating her ongoing worth. This asks family members to let go of the person they used to know and accept the person as she is now, but letting go and acceptance is a part of any relationship—even when no cognitive disorder exists.

When a patient no longer lives "now" but moves further back in time, even as far back as childhood, family mem-

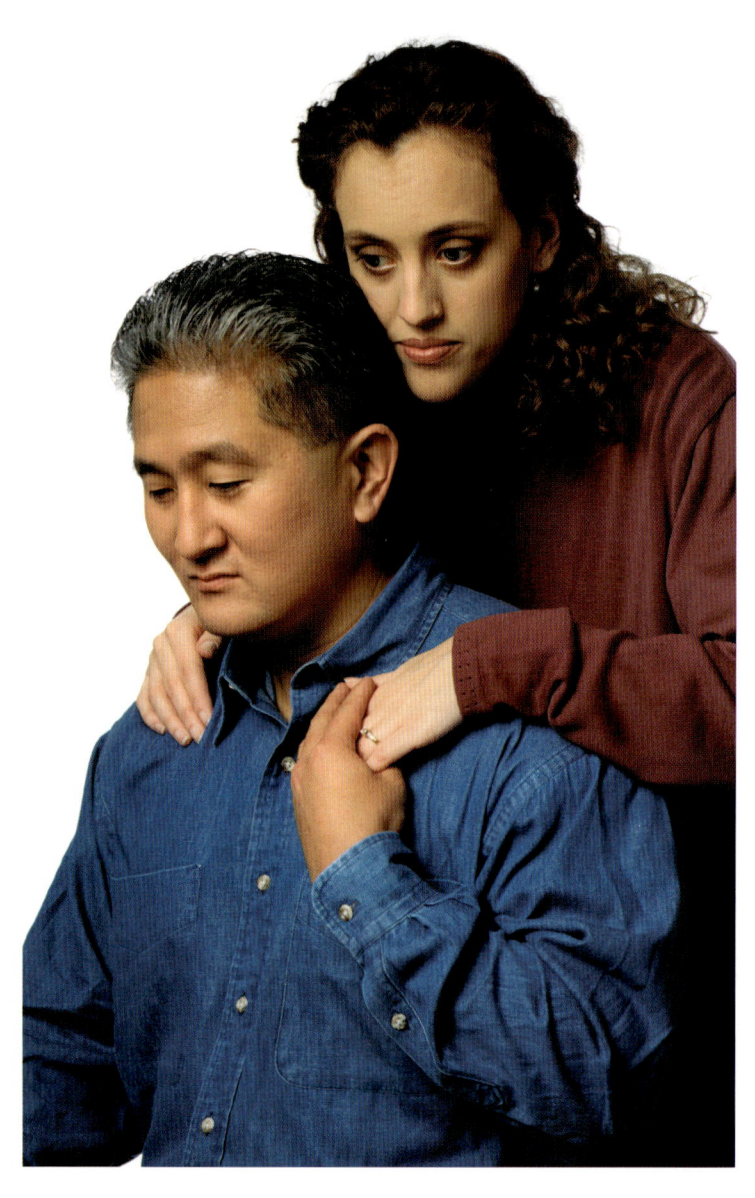

Memory loss doesn't need to interfere with loving relationships with family members.

bers are better off to move there also rather than try to bring the patient back to the present. Arguing and constant irritated reminders only cause agitation and anger. Many family members miss out on the joys left to experience with a loved one because they want things to be as they have always been. Acceptance and love give peace to everyone involved.

Family members also need to recognize the skills and strengths that the individual still possesses. A person with a cognitive disorder can no longer do many things. Depending at what phase she is at in her disorder, however, she will still be able to do many of the things she always did. A sense of responsibility and competence is important to self-worth. Living with someone whose mind is failing is much like living with a young child: both need to have tasks and responsibilities that are theirs, both need to feel included and valued, and both have much to contribute to the family's emotional quality of life.

Memory and other cognitive functions are essential components of life's daily tasks. As a result, memory loss is painful and debilitating. But we do not need memory to love or be loved.

FURTHER READING

Alterra, Aaron. *The Caregiver.* South Royalton, Ver.: Steerforth Press, 1999.

Castleman, Michael, Dolores Gallagher-Thompson, and Matthew Naythons. *There's Still a Person in There.* New York: G. P. Putnam's Sons, 1999.

Gorman, Jack M. *The Essential Guide to Psychiatric Drugs.* New York: St. Martin's, 1997.

Jones, Moyra. *Gentlecare.* Point Roberts, Wash.: Harley & Marks Publishing, 1999.

Mace, Nancy L., and Peter V. Rabins. *The 36-Hour Day.* Baltimore, Md.: Johns Hopkins University Press, 1999.

Shenk, David. *The Forgetting Alzheimer's: Portrait of an Epidemic.* New York: Doubleday, 2001.

FOR MORE INFORMATION

Alzheimer's Association
191 North Michigan Avenue, Suite 1000
Chicago, IL 60611-1676
800-272-3900
www.alz.org/

ADEAR Center
Alzheimer's Disease Education and Referral Center
P.O. Box 8250
Silver Springs, MD 20907
800-438-4380
adear@alheimers.org
www.alzheimers.org/adear

Alzheimer's Disease Cooperative Study (ADCS)
antimony.ucsd.edu/

Alzheimer's Disease and Research Center
The ALZHEIMER List and Alzheimer Digest
www5.biostat.wustl.edu/alzheimer/

Alzheimer's Research Forum
www.alzforum.org/home.asp

Alzheimer Society of Canada
20 Eglinton Ave. West, Suite 1200
Toronto, Ontario M4R 1K8
416-488-8772 or from Canada 800-616-8816
www.alzheimer.ca

126 | FOR MORE INFORMATION

Institute for Brain Aging and Dementia
www.alz.uci.edu/

National Institute of Mental Health
5600 Fisher's Lane, Rm. 7C02
Rockville, MD 20857
301-443-4513
www.nimh.nih.gov/

Publisher's Note:

The Web sites listed on this page were active at the time of publication. The publisher is not responsible for Web sites that have changed their address or discontinued operation since the date of publication. The publisher will review and update the Web sites upon each reprint.

INDEX

Alzheimer, Alois 17–18
amyloid plaques 17
antidepressants 32, 35, 100–104
antipsychotics 38–40, 77
anxiety 40, 42, 52

barbiturates 42
benzodiazepines 43, 56
brain 55, 58
brain cells 15, 17, 18

central nervous system 14
cerebral cortex 18
cognitive enhancers 60–63, 68, 69, 100

delirium 15
dementia 13–18, 20, 21, 28, 68
depression 31–34, 52
dopamine 21, 40

FDA 41, 73, 117

genes 19

herbal therapy 114–117
homeopathy 113
Huntington's Disease 14, 21, 40

imipramine 34–35
iproniazid 33

MAOIs 35–36, 71, 103
memory enhancers 43
mild cognitive impairment (MCI) 12, 14, 15, 96
multiple sclerosis 14

neurotransmitters 49, 52, 61

panic attacks 25, 31, 42
Parkinson's disease 14, 21, 87–93, 104
Prozac 38, 102–103
psychotherapy 110

serotonin 37, 40, 50, 52, 55, 56, 58
sleep 40–41
SSRIs 37–38, 55, 56, 70–72, 100–104
strokes 20

tacrine 27–28
tau 19

TCAs 37, 52, 73, 104

Valium 42
vitamins 112

BIOGRAPHIES

Sherry Bonnice lives with her husband and two children on a dirt road in rural Pennsylvania. Sherry has spent the last two years coediting quilt magazines and writing a quilt book. She has also written several books for two other Mason Crest series, Careers with Character and North American Folklore.

Carolyn Hoard received her master's degree in mental health counseling from Liberty University, Lynchburg, Virginia; she received her bachelor's degree in social work at Rochester Institute of Technology. Carolyn has been married 42 years to her husband, Jack, a hospital CEO; they have three children and six grandchildren. Carolyn was diagnosed with mild cognitive impairment, a possible precursor of Alzheimer's disease, in 2000.

Mary Ann Johnson is a licensed child and adolescent clinical nurse specialist and a family psychiatric nurse practitioner in the state of Massachusetts. She completed her psychotherapy training at Cambridge Hospital and her psychopharmacology training at Massachusetts General Hospital. She is the director of clinical trials in the pediatric psychopharmacology research unit at Massachusetts General Hospital and has a private practice as well.

Donald Esherick has spent seventeen years working in the pharmaceutical industry and is currently an associate director of Worldwide Regulatory Affairs with Wyeth Research in Philadelphia, Pennsylvania. He specializes in the chemistry section (manufacture and testing) of investigational and marketed drugs.